THE
COX-2
CONNECTION

THE
COX-2
CONNECTION

NATURAL BREAKTHROUGH TREATMENT
FOR ARTHRITIS, ALZHEIMER'S, AND CANCER

James B. LaValle, R.Ph., N.M.D., C.C.N.

HEALING ARTS PRESS
ROCHESTER, VERMONT

Healing Arts Press
One Park Street
Rochester, Vermont 05767
www.InnerTraditions.com

Healing Arts Press is a division of Inner Traditions International

*Note to the reader: This book is intended as an informational guide. The remedies,
approaches, and techniques described herein are meant to supplement, and not to be a
substitute for, professional medical care or treatment. They should not be used to treat a
serious ailment without prior consultation with a qualified health care professional.*

Library of Congress Cataloging-in-Publication Data

LaValle, James B.
   The Cox-2 connection : natural breakthrough treatment for arthritis,
Alzheimer's, and cancer / James LaValle B.
        p. cm.
   Includes bibliographical references and index.
   ISBN 0-89281-984-7
   1. Cyclooxygenase 2—Inhibitors. 2. Anti-inflammatory agents.
3. Alzheimer's disease—Treatment. 4. Antineoplastic agents. I. Title.
   RM405 .L38 2001
   615'.7—dc21

                                                    2001004627

Printed and bound in Canada

10 9 8 7 6 5 4 3 2

Text design and layout by Mary Anne Hurhula
This book was typeset in Janson with Avant Garde as a display face

Contents

Preface   vii

Part 1: The Problem and Treatment

1. An Overview of Inflammation   3

2. Understanding Your Anatomy: 18
   Muscles, Joints, and Bones

3. Common Inflammatory Disorders and Causes   30

4. Cox-2 Inhibitors: 50
   A Revolution in the Treatment of Inflammation

5. The Cox-2 Connection in Alzheimer's and Cancer   56

Part 2: What You Can Do

6. Natural Cox-2 Inhibitors   68
   and Other Natural Remedies

7. Current Treatment Options   87

8. A Smorgasbord of Ways to Manage Your Pain   109

Resources   146
Notes   154
Index   161

Preface

Society is moving faster than ever and people are faced with tough challenges every day. Some of the most uncomfortable experiences many of us are forced to cope with are muscle and joint pain and inflammation. Sometimes the muscle and joint problems are caused by activities such as jogging and working out in the gym and other times they are simply the result of age or a physical condition.

The bad news is that the longer we live and the more active we are, the more we are at risk for developing chronic pain and inflammation. But this is not a book about feeling bad. The information in this book should be used as a tool that you can use to become more energized and vital so you can deal effectively with the pain from inflammation that you are experiencing. In addition, this information can help you prevent other problems—both physical and emotional—that can be caused by these disorders if they remain untreated or are handled improperly.

Inflammation and chronic pain result from the wear and tear our bodies endure as we live longer. Our bones, muscles, tendons, and ligaments held up just fine for hundreds of thousands of years when life expectancy was about forty years. However, today, when most Americans can expect to live well into their seventies—and some into their eighties or nineties—these body parts begin to give way.

In medicine, much of pain management focuses on this new reality. Approximately 40 million Americans suffer from some form of arthritis. Within the next twenty years, that number will surge to 60 million. It is estimated that approximately 80 percent of people over age fifty suffer from some form of arthritis. And approximately 95 percent of those with arthritis have the form called osteoarthritis. The cost of arthritis to society is estimated to be well over $65 billion a year.

In our society, many people—especially baby boomers—are living more active lives than their parents did. They are working hard and playing hard. After a long day at the office, men and women head off to a strenuous evening at the health club. Vigorous athletic activity is a passion for many people. And women are now engaged in stressful activities that were once male-only sports, such as boxing and football. Joggers can be found running beside major highways outpacing cars caught in the rush-hour crawl, in suburban developments surrounded by spreading sprawl, and on long and winding rural roads. They are all engaged in these activities to increase their vitality, improve their health, and increase their longevity. These activities also appeal to those seeking to lower their stress levels. However, with such intense activity and increased longevity comes damage to many parts of the body, damage that can contribute to the development of inflammatory disorders.

There is some evidence that too much exercise can increase the risk of getting osteoarthritis. In a 1999 article in the *Journal of Rheumatology*, researchers reported that women who engaged in high levels of physical activity had a greater incidence of arthritis later in life. (Moderate exercise was not associated with the development of osteoarthritis.) Increased weight also puts a person at greater risk of developing osteoarthritis. Here exercise can help reduce weight and the risk of inflammatory disease.

Individuals seeking relief from pain and inflammation have many choices in today's medical environment. Over-the-counter and prescription non-steroidal anti-inflammatory drugs (NSAIDs); "nutraceuticals," such as glucosamine and chondroitin; and certain herbal supplements with anti-inflammatory activity are available for you and your health care provider to choose from.

The exciting news is that due to recent research, we understand the inflammatory response better than ever before, and we have come up with some pretty effective means to help people cope with it. Medical science is revolutionizing our insights into this problem. For example, a new synthetic "super aspirin" is now on the market under two different names: Celebrex and Vioxx. These two NSAIDs are called Cox-2 inhibitors. Their full story is not in yet, but they seem to hold great promise. Natural Cox-2 inhibitors may produce even greater benefits than the synthetic versions. Advances in pain management, through drugs and nondrug approaches, are improving the picture for those with inflammatory disorders.

The Cox-2 inhibitors Celebrex and Vioxx seem now to be revolutionizing physicians' prescribing habits. Cox-2 inhibitors are fast becoming some of the most prescribed pharmaceutical drugs on the market. Recent reports have one Cox-2 inhibitor outselling the anti-impotence medication Viagra™ (IMS Health, 1999), yet we may not have a complete understanding of the so-called Cox-2 inhibitors at this time.

Cox-2 inhibitors are agents that inhibit or reduce the effects of the enzyme cyclooxygenase 2, which is a key enzyme responsible for the inflammation response in the body. Inflammation follows when a pathway of biochemical events in the body is activated by various factors, including infection, trauma, oxidation due to mental or emotional causes (such as running late to an appointment, children coming home without school-books), environmental stresses (i.e., chemical exposure, heavy metals, pollution, drug liver metabolism, radiation), and other irritation. Inflammation is basically a nonspecific reaction of the immune system. Fortunately, there are natural Cox-2 inhibitors available for people to choose from if they are looking for a natural option (see chapter 6). These natural remedies, unlike the new synthetic versions that have been around for only a few years, have been used safely and effectively for thousands of years and can be very helpful for managing inflammation and pain—and they have a variety of other potential benefits. Cox-2 inhibitors may have uses for more than inflammation and pain—they may also benefit the body when used in the treatment of life-threatening illnesses such as Alzheimer's disease and certain cancers such as colorectal cancer.

Stress may be one of the key contributors to inflammation. Medical research has provided us with irrefutable physiological, neurological, and immunological evidence that has clarified many of the underlying issues involved in stress-related problems in general and the inflammatory response in particular. Stress is directly related to so many health problems, and inflammatory disease is one of them.

Centuries ago great physicians intuited that our emotions had a relationship to our physical state of well-being, but they could not prove the connection. One hundred years ago the physiologist Walter Cannon first described the "fight-or-flight" response. Fifty years ago, Hans Selye, M.D., had proved to his satisfaction that there is a direct link between mental stress and physical illness. Just over a decade ago psychologist Robert Ader, immunologist Nicholas Cohen, and others extended Selye's pioneering work and created a new medical discipline that is thriving today—psychneuroimmunology (PNI). PNI is making great contributions to our ability to effectively manage stress and related disorders.

Primary care physicians and other health care providers are coming to recognize more and more that many of the diseases (such as osteoarthritis and other chronic inflammatory diseases) their patients suffer from are directly related to stress that is managed poorly or not handled at all. We now know that chronic stress is toxic to almost every system in the body if it is not controlled. Chronic stress can lead to poor nutrition, substance abuse, crippling emotional disorders, life-threatening physical diseases, long-term illness, and a variety of destructive and self-destructive behavioral problems.

For example, studies have demonstrated that the high levels of cortisol present in people who are under constant stress poison the body. This hormone also increases your appetite and can contribute to your becoming overweight. Excess cortisol makes you more vulnerable to infections. It can even sometimes lead to fatal illness. Chronic stress poisons your system and destroys the natural state of balance in your body. In fact, because there is never any letup with chronic stress, it is the greatest threat to balance and health.

Many people resort to alcohol, drugs, cigarettes, excessive eating, or all of these habits in an attempt to manage their stress. At first, some of these behaviors seem to work. The person feels some relief. But after a time, they boomerang with a vengeance, leaving the individual with the original problem and a host of other difficulties such as addiction, to name but one.

Stress can result from any of the major challenges with which life presents us: birth or death; child rearing or the inability to have a child; marriage or divorce; the loss of a job or getting a new job. Caring for others can relieve stress, but it can also create stress if you do not care for yourself at the same time. Medical illness can result from stress, but disease can also increase your stress levels.

The answers and solutions are available. It is up to you to learn about them and put them to use in your daily life. Your life is in your hands. This book can help you learn how to prevent, alleviate, and even eliminate pain and the inflammatory disorders that may be part of your life—including arthritis, tendonitis, fibromyalgia, food allergies, and gout among others. But more, it can help you create a life of pleasure and creativity, one that today may seem beyond your wildest dreams. It is within your power to do so—starting right now.

Part 1

THE PROBLEM AND TREATMENT

1

An Overview
of Inflammation

Too often, many of us don't pay enough attention to our health. Our lives are so busy and we have barely enough time to devote to a job, a relationship, children, pets, finances, and so on. However, sometimes a health problem arises that catches and keeps your attention. You can't ignore it and function properly, so you are forced to do something to take care of yourself. Inflammatory disorders, and the pain and discomfort associated with their symptoms, are in this category. When they occur, you can't hide from them.

Fortunately, most symptoms of inflammatory disorders respond to a wide range of treatments. And there are effective solutions for even the most serious problems. It is important, though, to see a physician or other health care professional to obtain the correct diagnosis of your condition and to find the proper treatment.

The goal of this book is to help you understand the many different types of inflammatory disorders that can affect your muscles and joints and to learn what choices and options are available for the treatment of these conditions.

WHAT IS INFLAMMATION?

The most common symptoms of inflammation are swelling, redness, a sensation of heat at the affected tissue, and pain. The inflammation may be caused by a physical injury, a chemical irritation, or infection.

When the tissues of your body are damaged, specialized cells known as mast cells release a chemical called histamine. Although other chemical substances in the body are known to be involved in the inflammatory response, most experts agree that histamine is responsible for most of the symptoms of inflammation.

The redness you see and the heat you feel occur when histamine increases the blood flow to the damaged tissues. Histamine also causes the capillaries to become leaky. As a result, fluid seeps out of them and into the surrounding tissues, causing localized swelling. The pain that you feel is caused when nerve endings are stimulated by the inflammatory chemicals your body is producing.

When inflammation occurs, there is usually an accompanying accumulation of white blood cells. Thee cells, which are produced by your immune system, are attracted by the inflammatory chemicals. White blood cells have a twofold function: They help to destroy any invading foreign bodies and they help to repair damaged tissue.

Inflammation, in and of itself, is not a disorder. In fact, it is part of the body's self-regulating healing process. It is an essential part of your body's response to injury or infection.

THE ROLE OF PROSTAGLANDINS IN INFLAMMATION

Prostaglandins are messengers that the body produces to help regulate function. They play a key role in inflammatory disorders, and, for our purposes, a more important one than histamines. Prostaglandins are hormonelike substances. They have a number of functions in the body, among them to change the diameter of blood vessels and raise body temperature. Prostaglandins also play a vital role in blood clotting.

The body produces prostaglandins in response to injuries such as burns, sprains, strains, and breaks. The release of these substances causes redness, swelling, and inflammation. However, sometimes inflammation is an inappropriate response on the part of your body. This occurs in rheumatoid arthritis, for example, and in other autoimmune disorders.

Most of the major pain relievers available today—aspirin, ibuprofen, naproxen, and ketoprofen—reduce inflammation and are called nonsteroidal anti-inflammatory drugs (NSAIDs). The popular drug acetaminophen *does not* reduce inflammation and is a different kind of chemical.

NSAIDs all block the production of an enzyme in the body that is essential to the creation of prostaglandins—cyclooxygenase. This effect is important in the pain-relieving activity of the NSAIDs, but it is a double-edged sword. Prostaglandins help protect the digestive tract from the harmful effects of stomach acid. Because NSAIDs reduce the body's production of prostaglandins, they can cause gastrointestinal problems such as gastric ulcers (both peptic and intestinal), and intestinal bleeding.

It is claimed that the newest type of NSAIDs—known as the Cox-2 inhibitors—do not produce these adverse effects, but the full story on this class of drugs will be revealed only over time as millions of Americans take this expensive alternative to the older NSAIDs, which have been on the market for decades, or, in the case of aspirin, for a century. In fact, it was recently revealed to consumers that the chronic use of these common agents for pain and inflammation can lead to liver or kidney disorders, especially when combined with regular alcohol intake. For all the great science and research that goes on in the area of modern drug therapy, we simply do not know the long-term effects on the body of these very powerful and isolated chemical compounds.

EXTERNAL AND INTERNAL FACTORS INVOLVED IN INFLAMMATORY DISORDERS

Practitioners of Western medicine are increasingly becoming aware that when it comes to the health of the *whole* person, body and mind—the "bodymind"—it is usually not a choice of either/or; rather it is a matter of both/and. Proper diagnosis of health conditions must take into account both the endogenous and exogenous factors that may be involved in the onset of illness. The interplay between the two will determine the choice of treatment.

Endogenous factors are those that come from within the body. For example, a biochemical imbalance in the body may trigger an inflammatory response with no stimulus from the outside involved. *Exogenous* factors are those that come from outside. A splinter may cause inflammation in the affected area, or overexercise may cause an inflammation of a joint.

Your doctor's diagnosis of what brought on the inflammation will guide him or her in selecting the right treatment. However, even if a drug or natural product seems to be the proper way to manage the problem, there are other forms of intervention that are based not on the chemistry of a substance but on the interconnected functions of important systems of the human bodymind. A new medical discipline—psychoneuroimmunology (PNI)—has developed recently and is based on a new understanding of these functional interconnections.

Before we discuss the major types of inflammatory disorders, let's look at how some of these relevant systems work and see how they may relate to findings made in the field of PNI. The practical implications for treating and preventing disease will become evident.

THE IMMUNE SYSTEM, THE AUTONOMIC NERVOUS SYSTEM, AND PSYCHONEUROIMMUNOLOGY (PNI)

Your immune system plays a vital role in the body's ability to bounce back from the adverse effects of physical illnesses and emotional problems. Much of our new understanding of the interplay among the immune system, nervous system, and brain developed from the insights of the new discipline of PNI. This exciting information is the foundation for many of the recommendations for ways to treat the conditions (and alleviate their symptoms) that you will find in part two of this book.

Although Hippocrates, "the father of Western medicine," had recognized the mind-body connection thousands of years ago, it was not until 1991 that this reality was acknowledged by mainstream American medicine in an article that appeared in one of the medical establishment's most prestigious publications, the *New England Journal of Medicine*. The article recognized a correlation between psychological stress and susceptibility to infection with the common cold. A breach had been made in the wall that, for much of Western medicine, still kept the mind and body separate.

A lot has changed in the decade since that paper was published. For example, in the spring of 2000 a leading physician turned down an offer to be the editor in chief of *The New England Journal of Medicine*. Why did she decline to accept such an honored position? She chose instead to write a book on *alternative medicine*! Nearly 50 percent of Americans now see an alternative or complementary health provider (although 70 percent of these people don't tell their doctors), many major hospitals now have complementary care clinics, and most conventional medical schools now teach students about complementary approaches to health and healing.

Although these changes may seem to have occurred almost overnight, they were a long time coming and were the result of a groundswell of people in the United States who sought treatment from complementary practitioners underneath the very eyes of the established medical community. Along with recognizing the value of healing traditions from other cultures, the discipline of PNI has played a large role in helping to reshape American medicine and bridge the value of ancient principles of healing and health with the modern science–based aspects of health and healing.

In the 1970s psychologist Robert Ader and immunologist Nicholas Cohen performed a landmark experiment. In their animal study, the researchers gave rats an immunosuppressant drug along with saccharin-flavored water.

To their amazement, after some time, the saccharin-flavored water alone had the same effect on the rats as did the powerful immunosuppressant drug. Somehow, the immune system of the experimental animals had learned to associate the sweetened water with the effects of the potent chemical. The implication of their 1975 study was that the brain had the capacity to have a direct influence on immunity.

For hundreds of years, medical literature has included anecdotal reports suggesting that powerful emotional states were linked with such conditions as cancer, heart disease, ulcers, autoimmune disease, and allergies. But there were no Western-style clinical studies that proved this apparent link scientifically and definitively. However, an avalanche of credible scientific research followed the findings of Ader and Cohen, and many researchers have discovered a wide range of connections between the brain and the immune system.

A Brief Look at the Immune System

The immune system is composed of organs that are also called the lymphoid organs. They were given this name because they produce *lymphocytes*, the white blood cells that are an integral part of the immune response.

Lymphocytes are first produced in the bone marrow. Some lymphocyte—called T-cells—mature in the thymus gland, where they develop the ability to recognize the body or the self from what is foreign to the body. These white blood cells travel throughout the body, helping to fight off foreign organisms such as bacteria and viruses. Large amounts of lymphocytes are found in the spleen and the lymph nodes. They are poised and ready to go into action defending the body at a moment's notice. Scientists have discovered that the immunological organs—the thymus, lymph nodes, bone marrow, and spleen—are connected by nerve cells that act as pathways over which the brain and the central nervous system can influence the body's immune system.

Western scientists have come to recognize the interconnectedness of physical systems that were formerly believed to act autonomously and independently of one another. For example, it is now known that chemical messengers that were once thought to affect only nerve cells also have an effect on immune system cells. And it has been discovered that nerve cells react to chemicals produced by the immune system. In effect, these two systems can "talk" to each other. Further research has demonstrated that the nervous system connects the brain to the organs of the immune system and that the brain directly influences the production of immune system cells. These discoveries, along with many others, have formed the foundation of the new discipline of PNI.

The immune system is multifaceted and powerful. The immune response is a defensive reaction of the body to invasion by microorganisms, cancer cells, transplanted material, or other foreign bodies—substances not recognized as being a normal body component. Basically, the immune response consists of the production of antibodies, immunoglobulins, and lymphocytes, along with some other substances, that act to destroy invading materials, called antigens.

In addition to protecting the body, the immune system plays an important role in controlling cancer. It is also responsible for the rejection of organ and tissue transplants, allergy, and hypersensitivity.

Newborn children are protected against some forms of infection because they receive a kind of innate or natural immunity from their mothers, particularly through breast-feeding. This innate immunity acts quickly to defend the body; its protective actions are nonspecific. However, this innate immunity cannot protect the infant against all harm. The body, fortunately, has a second line of defense, called the adaptive immune system. This system fights off specific invading microorganisms and also has a *memory*. When the virus or bacterium is encountered again, it is recognized and the immune response is almost instantaneous. This acquired immunity can take days or weeks to develop. During this period, the newborn is vulnerable and years ago many babies died. Fortunately, better general health and nutrition, and effective immunizations, make it possible for more children to survive today.

The most important cells in the system are the lymphocytes. They are able to fight off threats to the body's integrity in many different ways. B-lymphocytes—or B-cells—produce circulating antibodies, which are tiny proteins that attack bacteria, viruses, fungi, and other foreign bodies (i.e., antigens). Antibodies are part of a family of proteins called immunoglobulins.

Somehow, each antibody is able to recognize the specific antigen it is to attack. The antibody will not attack any other invading organism. Antibodies fit antigens as specifically as a key fits into a lock. One antibody will fight the virus that causes the common cold, another the bacterium that causes pneumonia. Each B-lymphocyte produces only one specific antibody.

The T-lymphocytes—or T-cells—produced by the immune system attack invading organisms themselves. They do not produce antibodies to do the job for them. There are a number of different types of T-cells, each with a specific function. Cytotoxic T-cells and Natural Killer (NK) cells travel throughout the bloodstream. These T-cells and NK cells attach themselves to foreign bodies, destroying them by injecting them with toxic chemicals.

Each cytotoxic T-cell attacks only a specific type of foreign body. Some attack cancer cells, others go after cells infected with a virus. NK cells, on the other hand, can fight off a wide range of infectious microbes. There are two other types of T-cells—helper and suppressor cells—that play extremely important roles in the immune system. The helper cells are stimulants for the B-cells, prodding them to produce antibodies. After enough antibodies have been produced, the suppressor cells "turn off" the helper cells. Helper cells and suppressor cells "talk" to one another through a number of chemical messengers produced by the immune system, among them interferons and interleukins.

The Role of the Autonomic Nervous System

The *autonomic nervous* system controls the involuntary body functions, such as heart rate, digestion, and sweating. It affects the smooth muscles of the body (e.g., those in the airways and intestines) and not the striated muscles, which are under voluntary control. This network of nerves is divided into two parts: the sympathetic nervous system and the parasympathetic nervous system.

The *sympathetic nervous system* prepares the body for the "fight-or-flight" response. It quickens the heartbeat and breathing rate. The *parasympathetic system* has the opposite effect. It is more active in periods of relaxation. The two systems work together to help to create a state of balance in the body.

The sympathetic system is made up of two chains of nerves. They reach from the spinal cord to the organs and muscles they affect. The sympathetic nerve endings release neurotransmitters (i.e., epinephrine and norepinephrine) into the tissues. Also, this system stimulates the adrenal glands to release epinephrine into the bloodstream.

Among the most important actions of the sympathetic nervous system are strengthening and accelerating the heartbeat, widening the airways, dilating blood vessels in muscles and constricting blood vessels in the skin and abdominal muscles, decreasing digestive activity, dilating the pupils of the eyes, and producing the contractions in the urethra that produce the ejaculation of sperm in males.

The parasympathetic nervous system is also composed of two chains of nerves, one that passes from the brain and another that exits from the lower spinal cord. These nerves reach the same tissues, muscles, and organs as the sympathetic nerves. The nerves of the parasympathetic system release a neurotransmitter called acetylcholine. This chemical produces the opposite effects of epinephrine and norepinephrine. One function of the parasympathetic system helps to produce and maintain the erection of the penis in men who are sexually aroused.

The autonomic nervous system is inextricably connected to the experience of pleasure and anxiety in the body. Therefore, it plays a key role in many health-related problems, including inflammatory disorders.

Psychoneuroimmunology (PNI)

The word *psychoneuroimmunology* is composed of parts of three disciplines. *Psycho* represents the mind and/or brain; *neuro* stands for the neuroendocrine system, which consists of the nervous system and the hormonal system; and *immunology* refers to the immune system. The connections among these systems are not yet fully understood. However, it is becoming more and more obvious that there *are* real connections.

PNI research has exploded in recent years and investigators are studying how the physiological changes that occur in a body under stress or emotional distress can lead to physical problems such as heart disease, cancer, and diabetes.

There are three main areas of research in PNI that are providing evidence of the reality of the bodymind or "mindbody." First, physiological research looks into the connections between the brain and the other systems of the body in terms of biology and biochemistry. Second, a great deal of clinical work is being done that is demonstrating that mind-body approaches to health are quite successful in preventing and treating disease, as well as in alleviating symptoms. Third, epidemiological research—which studies large groups of people—is revealing links between certain psychological states and specific physical diseases in the general population.

Contemporary PNI physiological research can trace its roots back to Dr. Hans Selye's investigations into the physical effects of stress. The work of PNI investigators differs from mainstream medical research in many ways. For example, much mainstream research has focused on the relationship between cholesterol levels and heart disease. Billion-dollar blockbuster drugs have been developed based on this research. In contrast, PNI investigators look into the links between emotions and physical changes in the body. PNI research has trained its sights on the correlation between anger and heart disease. PNI researchers have also explored the link between repressed anger and arthritis as well as anger and lower-back pain. Mind-body medical solutions have been developed based on this body of work.

The fundamental question in mainstream biochemical research is, "Can a drug be developed that we can patent and sell?" The basic question for physiological PNI researchers is, "If emotional problems diminish the immune response, how does this relate to the onset of disease?"

In the early 1960s an epidemiologic study done for the U.S. Navy showed the relationship between physical illness and psychosocial factors. Sailors who had suffered serious emotional trauma (e.g., divorce, loss of job) were at a higher risk of becoming ill within a few months of those events. Recently, a substantial body of research has been developed that demonstrates that men and women who are socially isolated, or who have few meaningful social connections, are much more likely to become ill than are those who have close family ties and/or good friendships.

Clinical studies support the findings of the physiologists and the epidemiologists. One of the most powerful examples of this is the work done by Dr. David Spiegel of Stanford University, the author of *Living Beyond Limits*. When he began his research, which involved using hypnosis and relaxation in weekly sessions with a group of women who had advanced breast cancer, Dr. Spiegel was skeptical. The goal of his support group was simply to help these women cope with the consequences of their disease. However, when he looked at the survival rates of the women in his group, Dr. Spiegel was surprised to find that the women in the support groups lived eighteen months longer on average. A great deal of work has been done in this area at such prestigious institutions as Harvard, Stanford, UCLA, and Duke since Dr. Spiegel published his findings in the *Lancet* in 1989.

Ader, a psychologist at the University of Rochester School of Medicine and Dentistry, performed the breakthrough experiments that launched the field of PNI. Based on his work and the subsequent research in PNI performed over the past decades, scientists have described some of the essential connections among the mind-brain, the immune system, and the nervous system.

As was discussed earlier, Dr. Ader's key experiment with rats showed something startling—that the immune system can be influenced by conditioned response. In other words, the immune system has the power to *learn*. This amazing finding opened researchers' minds, and as they explored with open minds, they made further fascinating discoveries.

It was soon evident that the immune system can be influenced by many kinds of stress. Researchers discovered that chronic stress, or intense bouts of acute stress, impairs the immune system's ability to defend the body against outside challenges. It was later realized that hypnosis could be employed to influence the immune response. One of the experiments that proved this finding involved putting a chemical to which the research subject is allergic on both arms of the subject. While hypnotized, the person is told that the chemical will cause an inflammatory allergic reaction on only one arm. More often than not, the skin shows an inflammatory reaction on one arm only.

Later investigations indicated that psychosocial factors play an important role in the immune response as well. A wealth of papers have been published demonstrating that the susceptibility to a number of conditions—such as cancer, infections, and autoimmune disease—is affected by the impact of psychological and environmental conditions on a person's immune system. The progression of a disease, as well as an individual's response to treatment, can also be affected by psychosocial factors that impair the functioning of the immune system.

Researchers were surprised to find that there are nerve endings in the tissues of the immune system that connect the central nervous system to the bone marrow and the thymus as well as to the spleen and the lymph nodes. The cells of the immune system are produced in the bone marrow and thymus and are stored in the spleen and lymph nodes. These nerve connections show that the brain, central nervous system, and immune system are intimately interconnected.

Additional PNI research has proved that the brain closely monitors the activities of the immune system and can play an important role, both in altering the immune response and in initiating a response through the central nervous system.

Changes in the levels of the stress hormones and neurotransmitters in the body also alter the immune response. And the body's immune system can change the amount of these chemicals that are produced by the body. Researchers have also learned that lymphocytes—the key cells in your immune system—respond to the body's hormones and neurotransmitters. Lymphocytes are affected by endorphins (the body's natural opiates) and a wide range of hormones. In addition, it has been demonstrated that lymphocytes can also produce hormones and transmitters. Further, lymphocytes that are actively engaged in defending the body from a bacterium, virus, or other foreign body produce two kinds of substances—interferons and interleukins—that allow the immune system and the central nervous system to communicate with each other.

Drug research has also proved that psychoactive drugs have an effect on immune functioning, as do substances that are widely abused in our society, such as alcohol, nicotine, marijuana, cocaine, and heroin. In general, these drugs suppress the immune response. Lithium, the drug used to treat manic depression, has also been shown to alter the body's immune response.

The wealth of information that has been gathered through PNI research has radically changed the views of many Western medical researchers and physicians. It has demonstrated to them, through Western-style laboratory tests and human clinical studies, what has long been known in other healing traditions—that everything in the living organism is interconnected.

Until Ader's experiments, most scientists, researchers, and physicians in the West believed that the immune system, the brain, and the central nervous system were separate entities, not connected physically in any way and unable to have an effect on one another. At first, even Ader could not accept his discovery. He began to work with an immunologist, Cohen, and their efforts extended and deepened Ader's original findings. Over the ensuing years, their work has been repeated successfully worldwide.

As impressive as the research in PNI is, it is not the only discipline providing evidence for the intimate connections among brain, mind, emotions, health, and disease. Whereas PNI focuses on the immune system, new research shows that emotional distress and stress affect other systems as well, such as the circulatory and the digestive systems, frequent sites of inflammatory disorders. Psychological factors also affect the way we perceive the symptoms of illness, such as pain. And how severely we perceive these symptoms can have a profound effect on our daily lives. For example, two people may have the exact same type of lower-back pain or arthritis, yet one is crippled by the pain and the other functions quite well. Psychological factors can alter one's perception of pain and either diminish or improve the quality of life. There is also evidence that psychological factors can improve the quality of life for people with life-threatening conditions such as cancer.

The world's great healing traditions have known of the unity of the bodymind for millennia. It is one of the fundamental realities of their worldview and medical practice. At a recent international conference, a member of the audience asked the Dalai Lama's personal physician to speak about his views on the relationships among body, mind, and soul. Through a translator, the physician replied, "I don't understand the question." It is only Western medicine that has split the unitary organism into separate entities called body and mind or body and soul. Since such a splitting or duality does not exist in the Eastern worldview, the healer could not even understand what was meant by the question. This duality began 300 years ago with the philosopher Descartes and is deeply entrenched in our way of thinking. But it could not be more foreign to many other cultures.

It is now clear that the long-held belief in the dualities between the body and the mind, the mind and the brain, and the soul and the body are illusions. There is but one unitary organism and we are just learning how it functions. It has been quite difficult for mechanistic Western medicine to let go of this duality, but today, at the beginning of the twenty-first century, it seems that this crucial change is taking root. American medicine is being transformed, in part by the results obtained through PNI research and clinical trials, in part by the influence of other medical approaches (e.g., Ayurvedic medicine, traditional Chinese medicine, homeopathy, energy medicine), and in part by the demands of the public for improved health care through a combination of the best of conventional and the best of complementary medicine.

You will find that many of the self-care techniques recommended in part two of this book are based on the new insights gained from PNI and on the ancient insights achieved through millennia of healing experiences in other traditions.

PROMISING NEW RESEARCH

The most intensive research in managing the symptoms of inflammatory disorders is being carried out by the major pharmaceutical companies, which are eagerly seeking to develop the next blockbuster drugs, such as today's Cox-2 inhibitors. Drug treatment will always play a big role in our society, with its search for a quick cure and its "pill-for-every-ill" mentality.

In addition, many companies in the natural products industry are involved in exciting research and development that is bringing a number of new natural remedies to the market. These medicines have great potential to relieve pain and alleviate symptoms without the serious adverse effects that come with some of the powerful pharmaceuticals used for these conditions. In addition, may natural remedies fight inflammation in the same way as the new Cox-2 inhibitors, without the problems associated with synthetic drugs.

Increasing numbers of patients (and health care professionals too) are recognizing the value of complementary medicine in managing inflammatory disorders. Mind-body approaches, such as meditation and various relaxation techniques, are also showing great usefulness in helping to prevent, alleviate, and even eliminate these problems. More and more HMOs, health insurance companies, and other third-party payers are offering complementary medical care to their customers because they recognize the effectiveness of these modalities.

The National Center for Complementary and Alternative Medicine, one of the institutes within the National Institutes of Health, is undertaking a wide range of research at its regional centers. The center is also funding many independent researchers throughout the United States. Today, differing medical worldviews—which were until recently antagonistic to one another—are being combined into a new integrative approach to health care.

A "WHAT-YOU-CAN-DO" OVERVIEW

At first you may wonder how questions about worldviews or medical philosophies relate to preventing, alleviating, and eliminating inflammatory disorders. These are not ivory-tower questions. How a healer sees the world shapes his or her practice. What a researcher believes to be true can determine what he or she discovers in research or clinical trials. The application of the knowledge compiled by researchers all across the world can be of great value to you. This collective wisdom forms the basis for most of the recommendations that are made in part two of this book, which gives you information about many different ways to cope with these conditions. Following are the major areas that will be covered.

Drug Treatment

There are more drugs available to treat inflammation than ever before. The mainstays of drug treatment are the various anti-inflammatory agents that are now widely available as prescription drugs and as over-the-counter products. These drugs may be helpful for many people when properly used. The benefits and risks of drug therapy for inflammation will be discussed in detail later.

Aspirin (salicylic acid) is usually the first anti-inflammatory drug tried, unless an individual is allergic to aspirin or has another reason for avoiding it. Aspirin is quite effective in reducing inflammation and it is also relatively inexpensive. Acetaminophen (e.g., Tylenol) is also usually effective in relieving pain.

Other NSAIDs can also be effective, such as ibuprofen (Advil, Motrin), naproxen (Aleve), and ketoprofen (Actron, Orudis KT). As mentioned before, a new type of NSAID, called Cox-2 inhibitors, is now available. This class of drugs seems to cause fewer gastrointestinal side effects. Other drugs are used less frequently in less common situations and they will be covered in part two.

Drug therapy is not the only form of treatment available. Frequently, people find they can tolerate their symptoms as they learn to use one or a number of approaches to managing their condition.

Natural Remedies

Many herbs and other nutritional supplement products can be helpful in the treatment of inflammatory disorders. More and more people are turning to this form of medicine.

Exercise

Physical activity is a good thing and essential to your health. But as with almost everything in life, you can have too much of a good thing, or engage in it in the wrong way or at the wrong time. Exercise can help relieve pain at times, but it may contribute to inflammation and the onset of pain at other times. Sensible suggestions for how and when to exercise will be discussed later in the book.

Nutrition

Foods sometimes can cause biochemical problems in the body or exacerbate existing conditions, such as inflammation. Natural remedies and dietary supplements can help to bring the body back into balance biochemically. In addition, a lack of proper nutrients can diminish the effectiveness of treatment. A healthy nutritional regimen can be helpful in resolving some cases of inflammatory disorder. Stress is frequently associated with inflammatory problems and can deplete the body of essential nutrients. A healthy diet is especially important at such times. And an inadequate diet can sometimes bring on the symptoms of physical and emotional stress in certain individuals, clouding the clinical picture.

Mind-Body Techniques

The field of mind-body medicine has gained increasing acceptance in the past decade and offers much that is of great value to anyone seeking to cope with a wide range of medical problems. Many effective techniques to deal with pain and illness are discussed in detail later in the book.

Lifestyle Changes

Sometimes we can be our own worst enemies and our daily habits (e.g., smoking, drinking too much, lack of exercise, overexercising) can be the cause of many of the health problems we experience. And, unfortunately, it is frequently difficult for many people to see the connection between their habitual behavior and their emotional and physical distress. For example, many people work out at the gym or have a few drinks to unwind. However, these activities may at times contribute to health problems (e.g., joint inflammation and gout). Fortunately, inflammatory disorders can sometimes respond positively to changes in lifestyle and these will be discussed in part two as well.

Inflammatory disorders appear to be on the rise and will probably continue rising as baby boomers enter their fifties and sixties. These conditions can dramatically decrease your quality of life—but they do not have to! There are many effective ways of handling them. We will take a closer look at these disorders. First, let's look at the body and its functions when relating to inflammation.

2

Understanding Your Anatomy: Muscles, Joints, and Bones

THE BODY'S MUSCLES

Your body is able to move with great flexibility because it is supported by a framework of muscles, joints, and bones. Both the movement of your body as a whole in the outside world and the movement of the organs inside your body are dependent on muscles that are made of tissues that have the ability to contract. Muscle tissue is made of tiny filaments. These filaments go into action when they are stimulated by nerve impulses. The movement of the filaments produces either contraction or relaxation. It is because of this movement that a muscle is able to do its job.

Some muscles, such as the ones in your arms and legs, are under your conscious control. These muscles contract only when you decide to undertake an action, such as pick up a tool in the garage or reach for something in the kitchen cabinet. Today it is believed that the brain sends signals through the nervous system to the muscles involved, so that they either contract or expand, depending on the activity involved. These muscles are called the *voluntary muscles.*

The other muscle group consists of the *involuntary muscles.* The most easily recognizable muscle in this group is the heart. Other involuntary muscles are involved in such body processes as digestion, respiration, and sexual functioning. The involuntary muscles perform their functions without an individual being aware of them (unless something is going wrong) and without being under conscious control.

The muscles are attached to bones at each end by tendons, which are bands of connective tissue. Similar tissues called ligaments surround joints and connect one bone to the other.

There are three different types of muscle in the body: skeletal, smooth, and cardiac.

Skeletal Muscle

The body contains more than 600 voluntary muscles as part of its skeletal muscle system. The largest part of the musculature is composed of these skeletal or voluntary muscles. The skeletal muscles are divided into a number of different types depending on the kind of action the muscle performs. *Extensor muscles* open joints and *flexor muscles* close them. *Adductor muscles* pull parts of the body in, while *abductor muscles* move them outward. A *levator muscle* raises a body part and a *depressor muscle* lowers it. And *constrictor* or *sphincter muscles* close body orifices or surround them.

Skeletal muscles, which are made of groups of muscle fibers, are found in the body in orderly arrangements. A small muscle, for example, may contain only a few fiber bundles. In contrast, the major muscles are composed of hundreds of bundles of fibers. And the muscle fibers themselves are built from even smaller structures called myofibrils. The basic units of the myofibrils are two microscopic filaments, actin and myosin. These two proteins are extremely important because they control muscle contraction.

According to present theory, the voluntary muscles are under the control of the brain. Each muscle fiber is connected to a nerve ending that receives impulses from the brain. The muscle is stimulated and put into action by a chemical secreted by the nerve called acetylcholine, a neurotransmitter.

When acetylcholine is released, a whole chemical and electrical cascade is set into motion. Sodium, potassium, and calcium ions cause the myosin filaments to slide over the actin filaments, and this results in a muscle contraction. Each muscle also contains specialized nerve fibers that measure the force of the contraction. There is also a parallel set of fibers in the tendons that register the stretch of the muscle. All of this information is transmitted to the brain and has an impact on muscle activity.

Chemical changes in the fluids surrounding muscle cells have an effect on the activity of the skeletal muscles. For example, if the potassium level drops, the muscles may become weak. Or if there is a decrease in calcium, there may be muscle spasms.

Smooth Muscle

Smooth muscles are involved in the functioning of the internal organs. These movements are exemplified by the contractions of the uterus during childbirth and by the movement of the intestines called peristalsis. Other organs also contain smooth muscles—for example, the bronchi of the lungs, the walls of blood vessels, and the bladder.

These muscles are made up of long, spindle-shaped cells. The cells are arranged in two layers in the hollow organs. The outer layer is longitudinal and the inner layer is circular. The contraction of the smooth muscles works in the same way it does in the skeletal muscles.

The nerves of the autonomic nervous system connect with the smooth muscles, leaving them outside the bounds of conscious control. The nerves actually penetrate into the muscle, where they branch out. Neurotransmitters are released from these branches and they initiate the contractions of the smooth muscles.

Hormones also affect the functioning of the smooth muscles, as do changing levels of oxygen and acid in the surrounding bodily fluids.

Cardiac Muscle

This type of muscle is found in only one place—the heart. This unique muscle is called the myocardium. It is able to contract in a rhythmic manner over 100,000 times a day, enabling it to send blood throughout the body. Structurally, cardiac muscle is similar to skeletal muscle. As with the smooth muscles, cardiac muscle is stimulated by the autonomic nervous system, hormones, and the effects of stretching muscle fibers.

To work efficiently, the muscles of the heart must operate in a regular manner. The arrangement of the muscle fibers in the heart allows for the contractions to be rapidly transmitted from one fiber to another. Specialized cardiac muscle cells carry out this vital task.

THE BONES: YOUR SUPPORT SYSTEM

There are 206 bones in your body and most of them provide support for the other parts of the body. Some bones also play a protective role. The skull, for example, protects the brain from harm. The vertebrae of the spine protect the nerves of the spinal column. The pelvis, at the base of the abdomen, shields the bladder and portions of the genital tract. And the rib cage guards the heart and lungs as well as the organs in the upper abdominal area of your body—the liver, kidneys, stomach, and spleen.

We often think of bones as static structures, yet bones are as alive as any other part of the body. Bone tissue is made up of living cells just as are the eyes, the skin, the lungs, and almost all other parts of the body. These cells are housed in collagen, a protein that is saturated with phosphorus and calcium. The collagen stores and supplies essential minerals that the bones need to stay strong and healthy. Bone tissue is made up of tiny cylinders of organic material that contain many minerals, predominantly calcium and phosphorus. A great deal of the strength of bone comes from these cylinders.

In addition, deep inside some of the bones is the marrow. Inside the marrow, specialized cells manufacture blood cells.

The bones of the skull are joined by sutures, which are immovable connective fibers. Most of the other bones are connected by what are commonly called joints. The joints are like hinges that connect certain bones, allowing them to move in relation to each other. The knees and the elbows are examples of joints where bones connect.

Bones come in two main shapes—flat and long. The plates of the skull and the vertebrae are examples of flat bones. The thigh bones and arm bones are examples of long bones. Despite external differences, the internal structure of bones is basically the same. Blood vessels run through the bones and are surrounded by nerves. The bones in the body come together to form joints.

There are a number of different kinds of joints in the body. For example, the spinal column is composed of individual vertebrae, each of which can move only slightly. However, these slight movements give the spine enough flexibility so that a person can bend the back to a considerable degree.

The joints of the fingers are known as hinge joints. They allow movement in one plane only—that is, backward and forward. The elbow joints move in the same way. A more versatile type of joint is called the ball-and-socket joint. The shoulder is an example of this. This kind of joint allows movement in nearly any direction. Because of the ball-and-socket joint, you can turn, twist, and bend your arm. The actions of the arms involve a combination of all the movements allowed by these different types of joints.

Joints are complicated structures bound together by fibrous bands called ligaments. And within each ligament is a capsule composed of fibrous tissue that surrounds the joint. Ligaments stabilize and strengthen the joints, permitting movement in certain directions. At the point where the ends of the bones meet, all the surfaces are covered by smooth, flexible cartilage.

All of the components of a joint work together to produce movement that is harmonious and balanced and that causes no harm to the body. When you look into the workings of the body, you cannot help but be deeply impressed by the magnificence of life. This can be seen in something as simple as the taking of a single step.

When you bend your knee to take a step, your hamstring muscles, which are on the back of the thigh, contract. They then pull in the lower leg and bend the knee. Simultaneously, the quadriceps muscles on the front of the thigh relax. This allows the knee to bend. Inside the knee, friction is minimized by synovial fluid and cartilage. The five ligaments around the bone help keep the skeletal structure properly aligned. Cushioning is provided by structures called bursa at the knee and other parts of the body.

So much activity goes into such a simple thing as taking one step. The body functions in a coordinated, balanced manner when it is in a healthy state.

THE MUSCULOSKELETAL SYSTEM

The bones and muscles work together in what is called the musculoskeletal system. Many inflammatory disorders involve this system intimately, so it's helpful to have a basic idea of what it is and how it works.

In general, skeletal muscles are attached to two or more bones. The muscles of the body do not usually work individually but rather in coordinated groups. For example, when one muscle contracts, a related muscle usually relaxes. At the same time, other muscles in the same part of the body act to stabilize the nearby joints. When a muscle contracts, the bones to which it is attached move.

The muscles in the head and neck have many roles to play. The contraction of these muscles produces our facial expressions, communicating joy, sorrow, anger, fear, and other emotions. The muscles also allow the head to move in many directions. In addition, head and neck muscles make it possible for us to swallow and to speak.

The abdominal muscles are a large group with a variety of actions. These muscles are essential to regular breathing. They also help balance the muscles around the spine when you are lifting things. And the abdominal muscles help to keep the abdominal organs safely in place.

The muscles in the arms are found primarily at the shoulder and below the elbow. The muscles in the forearm are connected to the wrist and fingers by long tendons. The muscles in the legs are among the most powerful in the body. They are anchored solidly in a number of points, particularly at the pelvis.

The bones in the male and female skeleton are basically the same, although usually those of a woman are somewhat smaller. The pelvis is an important exception. A woman's pelvis is generally wider than a man's. It also has a larger space in the middle, which allows the head of a baby to pass from the uterus through the pelvis at birth.

Musculoskeletal Disorders

Problems with the musculoskeletal system are major causes of both physical disability and chronic pain. And the inflammatory response is associated with both types of health problems.

The body is designed to move and movement is essential to health. However, over long periods of time, the body can suffer from injuries or simply become worn out from overuse, both of which can result in inflammation. Until relatively recently, fifty to one hundred years ago, the average life expectancy for an American was between forty and sixty years. In the 1930s one of the reasons that age sixty-five was chosen as the age at which people could collect Social Security was that most people did not live to be sixty-five and therefore would not collect any benefits. Today, life expectancy for men and women in the United States is in the upper seventies and is continuing to rise. So it is not surprising that we are witnessing increased numbers of musculoskeletal disorders and related inflammation.

In addition, many more people—particularly aging baby boomers—are engaging in exercise programs designed to increase their vitality and longevity. Due to overexercise or working out improperly, many people are suffering injuries that result in inflammation.

It is quite common for bones, muscles, joints, tendons, and ligaments to become injured. These injuries can range from minor sprains and muscle pulls to more serious problems, such as dislocated shoulders, torn ligaments, and broken bones.

INFLAMMATION—NATURE'S RESPONSE

One of the most common natural responses to injury—be it the irritation of tissues or damage to muscles, joints, or bones—is inflammation. The most frequent symptoms of inflammation are swelling, redness, a sense of heat or warmth at the injured spot, and a loss of natural movement or functioning.

In medical lingo, *itis* at the end of a word indicates an inflammatory condition. For example, an inflammation of a joint is called arthr*itis*. An inflammation of a tendon is referred to as tendin*itis*. Inflammation may be confined to a small part of the body—localized in a joint, for example—or it may be widespread, as with an inflammatory disease like rheumatoid arthritis (RA).

Inflammation may be acute and pass quickly, such as the inflammation caused by a splinter. Or it may become chronic and last for a long period of time, as it does with certain immune responses, mineral deposits in the body, or with mechanical stress from continued use of an injured body part or overuse of a body part.

Inflammation because of injury to the musculoskeletal system must be distinguished from inflammation caused by an underlying disease process. For example, bone and joint infections can cause permanent disability if not identified and treated properly. And both benign and cancerous tumors can start in the bone; cancerous growths can spread to other parts of the body if undetected. Disorders of the metabolism or hormonal imbalances may also affect bones and joints. Osteoporosis and gout are two such examples.

Lab tests can sometimes provide helpful information, but usually such tests alone are not adequate. X rays of inflamed, painful areas are taken to help make a diagnosis. With X rays, physicians can determine whether or not there are any fractures, infections, or other serious problems causing the inflammation, other than an injury. In addition to X rays, CT scans and magnetic resonance imaging (MRI) may be needed to make a correct diagnosis of the problem and to determine proper treatment. MRI is very useful when investigating muscles, tendons, and ligaments.

Also, it may be necessary to take a sample of joint fluid to get a clear picture of what is taking place in the body. Examination of the fluid can reveal whether a bacterial infection is the source of the problem or if there are crystals present that would indicate the patient is suffering from gout.

Treatment varies with the type of musculoskeletal problem and its severity. Rest, immobilization with splints, painkillers, topical applications, and hot or cold compresses may all be helpful, alone or in combination. Effective treatment may require the efforts of physicians, physical therapists, occupational therapists, and physiotherapists all working together.

JOINT AND CONNECTIVE TISSUE DISORDERS

Diseases affecting the many components of the joints—muscles, bones, ligaments, and cartilage—are known as connective tissue diseases. These parts of the body contain large amounts of connective tissue. In addition, an autoimmune response, in which something triggers the immune system to attack the body's own tissues, may cause joint and connective tissue disorders.

Inflammation is a basic characteristic of both immune reactions and autoimmune reactions. With an appropriate immune response, inflammation is a healthy part of the body's self-healing efforts and it is short-lived. However, in the autoimmune response, inflammation may become chronic and persistent. This can result in damage to normal tissues. In rheumatoid arthritis, the autoimmune response damages the cartilage in the joints. The connective tissues near joints and elsewhere in the body can also become inflamed. Muscles, too, may suffer inflammation under these conditions.

Treatment of these conditions varies with the severity of the problem and the specific diagnosis involved. In the past, NSAIDs have been used to reduce inflammation of less serious conditions. However, more drastic measures may be required if the inflammatory process is affecting the pericardium surrounding the heart or the membrane around the lungs.

MUSCLE, BURSA, AND TENDON DISORDERS

If the body is to move properly and function normally, the muscles, bursa, and tendons must be healthy. As has been noted earlier, the muscles are connected to the bones by tendons, and when muscles contract, they move the bones to which they are attached. The bursas are fluid-filled sacs that act as cushions and reduce friction at the spots where muscles, tendons, and ligaments meet bone.

Overuse, injury, or infection can damage these parts of the body. Injury to these areas is characterized by pain and inflammation. Common conditions associated with these parts of the body are myositis (muscle inflammation), bursitis, tendinitis, and fibromyalgia syndromes, characterized by pain in the soft tissues, muscles, tendons, and ligaments.

COMMON PROBLEMS

The musculoskeletal system is quite susceptible to injury, perhaps more so than many other parts of the body. Muscles can be torn if pushed beyond their capacities, bones can be broken by extreme force, and the ligaments and tendons that bind bones at joints can be torn if the joint is forced into unnatural movements. These parts of the body frequently develop both acute and chronic damage, with resulting pain and inflammation.

Pulled Muscles

When muscles are overstretched, fibers tear. When this occurs, muscles contract and may also become swollen. If the damage is severe enough, the muscle may rupture or be torn completely. When a person experiences a muscle pull, pain is felt when the injury occurs. The affected muscle will not function properly until the injury heals. At first the muscle may feel tender and swollen. Later it may become stiff and painful.

Almost everyone will experience a muscle pull or strain at some time in his or her life, especially those who play sports or work out. In general, recovery is complete in a short period of time. However, a serious strain or tear may cause permanent damage if it is not treated properly. Recovery slows as people age, and older people can do greater damage than younger people can.

Sprains

When too much pressure is put on a joint, the ligaments holding the bones together may be stretched or perhaps even torn. This is commonly referred to as a sprain. The knees, ankles, and fingers are the joints most likely to experience sprains, but any ligament can be damaged.

A sprained ligament can still function, but usually only with pain. There may be swelling and discoloration of the skin in the affected area. If a sprain is extremely severe, with all the ligaments torn, the joint may be misshapen as well as swollen. Minor sprains present no great danger, but joints will weaken if the ligaments are frequently torn and stretched.

Severed tendons, fractures and broken bones, and dislocations are serious injuries that require immediate treatment at an emergency room, in a hospital, or by a physician.

Cramps

A cramp is a spasm in a muscle. Cramps can sometimes be quite painful. Nearly everyone will experience cramps at one time or another, usually as a result of sitting or standing too long, spending too much time in an uncomfortable position, or performing exercise at a level greater than usual. For some people, cramps occur in the middle of the night and they awaken in pain. Fortunately, the pain is short-lived and there is usually no underlying health problem that is causing the cramps.

Tendinitis

When the tissue that connects muscles to bones (i.e., tendons) is injured and becomes inflamed or torn, the area of the body that is affected becomes tender, painful, and swollen. Tendons heal more slowly than other parts of the body because the muscles are constantly in use. Also, very little blood reaches the tendons and this impairs healing.

Tendinitis usually heals within a few weeks. However, the pain may last for months. In older people, the pain may persist and even get worse over time. Overexertion in sports can produce tendinitis such as "tennis elbow" or "golfer's elbow." This condition also frequently affects the shoulders and heels.

Repetitive Strain Disorder

A membrane called the synovium covers some membranes, such as those of the fingers and thumbs. If the fingers are used in repetitive tasks, such as typing and assembly-line work, this membrane can become swollen, causing what is known as repetitive strain disorder or tenosynovitis. The area over the tendon may become tender and painful, and it may be difficult to straighten bent fingers.

Fibromyalgia

This condition is marked by pain and tenderness in the fibrous tissues deep within the muscles. There is no known cause for fibromyalgia, but it does seem to be related to emotional tension that causes muscles to tighten and knot. In this condition, although the muscles themselves are healthy, the person may feel pain and experience some swelling. People with fibromyalgia frequently suffer from back pain. This condition usually clears up on its own and requires only symptomatic treatment.

Back Pain

The backbone, or spinal column, is composed of more than thirty vertebrae that are connected by ligaments and flat, flexible disks that lie between the bones. The spinal column stretches from the skull to the buttocks and protects the spinal cord from damage. The outside of the disks is made of a fibrous substance that covers an inner substance that is like jelly in consistency. This structure makes it possible for the entire spine to move. However, the flexibility of the spine is limited and this contributes to much back pain.

The majority of backaches are called "nonspecific" because there is no obvious cause of the pain. Psychological factors, muscle strain, injury, and poor posture may all play a role in back pain, either singly or in combination. Nonspecific backache can be extremely painful and is one of the major causes of absence from work. This condition may interfere with daily life, but it usually heals without any treatment and there is no significant risk of complications developing.

Lower-back pain, coccygeal pain, and sciatica are the most common forms of back pain. Lower-back pain is centered in the small of the back and is usually caused by heavy lifting, moving furniture, overwork in the garden, or some other form of overexertion. Coccygeal pain is located at the base of the spinal column, near the coccyx. It is usually caused by falling on the buttocks or some other injury to that area. Some women suffer from this pain after childbirth. There are special pillows available to bring relief to those suffering from this form of backache. The pain from sciatica results from pressure on the sciatic nerve, which is the largest of all the nerves and branches out all through the legs and lower body. It is characterized by a burning pain that runs from the buttocks down the back of the thigh. Sometimes there is also tingling and/or numbness.

Bursitis

Bursas are soft sacs containing fluids that minimize friction between body parts that constantly rub against one another. These sacs are found predominantly near joints. If a bursa is injured or becomes irritated by pressure, it can become inflamed and swollen with fluid. This condition is called bursitis and it is quite common. The shoulders, the elbows, the kneecaps, the hips, the heels, and the base of the big toes are all areas of the body that are susceptible to bursitis.

Frozen Shoulder

With this condition, normal movement of the shoulder becomes impossible. This painful disorder that causes stiffness may start with something like bursitis or tendinitis, which can prevent a person from using the joint fully. The lack of use leads to more pain and a gradual weakening of the shoulder and further loss of function. If this condition is not treated, it will slowly worsen and leave the individual with an immobile shoulder. It is imperative to see a physician if this condition seems to be developing.

Inflammation regularly accompanies all of the disorders described above. Although the mainstay of treatment is drug therapy, particularly the use of prescription or over-the-counter NSAIDs, there are other methods for tackling these problems and their symptoms; they will be discussed in later chapters of this book.

This brief overview of how the body functions will help you to better understand how the treatments that are described in later chapters affect the body and why doctors and other health care providers recommend them.

3

Common Inflammatory Disorders and Causes

ARTHRITIS

Arthritis is the most common form of inflammatory disorder in the United States today. But it is not the only variety of inflammation from which people suffer. In this chapter, we will look at a range of conditions caused by inflammatory processes.

About 40 million Americans suffer from arthritis in one form or another, including 80 percent of those people over age fifty. With someone turning fifty every ten seconds in this country, it is easy to see the significance of the problem. Over the next two decades, 75 million members of the baby boom generation will develop this disorder, and it is expected that there will be nearly 60 million Americans whose lives will be impaired by some type of arthritis.

This disease appears to affect more women than men, with a prevalence rate of 60 percent for women. In addition to the incalculable human costs of arthritis, the economic costs are high. According to a National Institutes of Health Interview Survey, in the United States the total cost of arthritis is about $65 million a year. The indirect costs, such as lost wages, made up nearly 75 percent of this figure.

Arthritis is a complex disease that is not thoroughly understood, and treatment of this condition still leaves a lot to be desired. As a result, many patients become discouraged as one form of therapy after another leaves them still suffering. However, there are many things that you can do to help improve your situation. By learning as much as you can about arthritis, you can begin to take effective action that will bring symptomatic relief from pain and also improve other debilitating aspects of the condition, such as loss of physical mobility.

Signs and Symptoms

Symptoms of arthritis will depend upon the type of arthritis that is present. However, some general symptoms include:

- Stiffness
- Swelling in one or more joints
- Deep, aching pain in a joint
- Any pain associated with movement of a joint
- Tenderness, warmth, or redness in afflicted joints
- Fever, weight loss, or fatigue that accompanies joint pain

The more you know about arthritis, the more effectively you can take preventive measures to avoid many problems. For example, the more you know about the ups and downs of the course of the disease, the better you will be able to act to minimize the physical limitations it produces.

While it is important for you to take responsibility for your own health and learn as much as you can, it is just as important for your physician or health care provider to explain your course of treatment to you—what you are doing and why. If your doctor has you trying one drug after another, he or she needs to explain the rationale behind this. If you are using natural or herbal remedies, the health professional recommending these remedies needs to explain to you why you are using them. And if you are trying any of the many effective mind-body approaches, it will be of great help if the health professional you are working with explains the rationale of these therapies to you.

When possible, it is also of great value for a spouse, family members, or other people who share your life to learn about what you are going through. This will allow them to be more supportive.

How can education help you and those close to you? In a study published in the *Journal of Rheumatology* in August 1999, Canadian researchers reported that arthritis patients were better able to manage their disease if they received more information about it. The researchers worked with 252 patients, divided into two groups, who were receiving drug therapy for their arthritis. Fifty percent of the patients received extra educational information—a thirty-minute interactive computer session on the drug they were taking, an audiotape to listen to at home, and a booklet on the medication to take home and refer to when needed. The other 50 percent received only general information on the drug they were taking. The researchers found that 38 percent of those in the group that received more educational information found it easier to follow the treatment plan and to take the drug safely. The researchers also said that increased information appeared to improve the outcome of treatment.

OSTEOARTHRITIS (OA)

The most common form of arthritis is called osteoarthritis (OA). This condition is sometimes referred to as degenerative joint disease and about 20 million Americans suffer from it at any particular time. In fact, by the age of forty, there is X-ray evidence of the presence of OA in the weight-bearing joints (e.g., the knees and hips) in nearly 90 percent of men and women.

OA does not impact overall survival of those who suffer from it. (Other forms of arthritis do affect longevity.) But if there is severe OA in the spinal column, the hips, or the knees, this will greatly limit activity. OA can cause much pain and discomfort, resulting in a poor quality of life for some.

What Causes OA?

The main cause of primary OA is the breakdown of cartilage. This deterioration comes as a result of stress on the joints that can occur over decades. Obesity is a major contributor to this condition. Obesity not only increases the risk of developing OA, but it also increases the risk for all other types of arthritis. The Centers for Disease Control and Prevention has reported that in both men and women who are obese, there is a 30 percent increased risk of developing arthritis. A number of published studies suggest that there may also be genetic factors involved in the onset of OA. For example, genetic factors appear to have played a role in the development of OA of the hands and knees in 39 to 65 percent of female twins who were evaluated in a recent investigation.

The first change that occurs in the body with OA is a roughening of the articular cartilage. This part of the body contains a gel-like protein collagen that is predominantly water. Subsequently, OA causes this structure to become pitted and ulcerated. The surface of the structure loses its cartilage progressively.

OA most commonly occurs in the joints of the spine, fingers, knees, and hips. It can also affect the base of the thumb and the big toe. OA can appear in one part of the body, a few parts, or throughout most of the body; however, it only rarely affects the shoulders, wrists, elbows, and ankles.

Another form of OA—called secondary arthritis—may appear in almost any joint of the body. Secondary arthritis has a number of common causes. It may result from an injury or trauma, or it may be caused by the overuse of a particular joint over extended periods of time. Also, another form of arthritis, such as rheumatoid arthritis, may lead to the development of secondary arthritis.

After trauma or injury, the body can usually repair the affected area. However, this is more difficult when the body tries to repair cartilage. There is limited blood supply to cartilage and this impedes repair. In addition, the body does not have a very effective method for the regrowth of cartilage.

Let's look at one cause of secondary arthritis—the overuse of joints. Researchers have found that people whose work involved at least a half hour per day kneeling or squatting, or climbing over ten flights of stairs, were more than two and a half times more likely to develop OA in the knees than people who did not have to engage in such activity regularly.

Symptoms of secondary OA usually appear at earlier ages than do symptoms of primary OA. This is due to the more rapid deterioration of the cartilage that is caused by overuse of, or trauma to, the joints.

The first symptoms of OA, which usually appear between the ages of forty and fifty, are generally quite mild. You may experience stiffness in the morning. This stiffness does not persist for more than ten or fifteen minutes. Or you may experience mild pain when the affected joint is moved. This pain can get better or worse with motion, better from cold or warmth, and worse in damp or wet weather. Some people develop these early symptoms of OA but the disease does not progress any further. However, others find that the pain and stiffness increase in severity. As OA progresses, it has a negative impact on daily activities such as typing, walking, and climbing stairs.

Two common examples of later-stage OA involve the joints of the fingers. The medical term for knobby growths of the joints nearest to the fingertips is Heberden's nodes and such growths at the middle joints of the fingers are called Bouchard's nodes. The former are more common in women than in men and they seem to run in families.

Diagnosing OA

In order to diagnose OA, a thorough physical examination and complete medical history are required. It is only through these diagnostic procedures that it can be determined whether arthritis is present and which type it is. Similar symptoms may be caused by other medical problems and these two procedures will clarify the situation.

When taking a medical history, a physician will ask you some standard questions to help identify whether arthritis is the cause of the problems you are experiencing. For example, your doctor will ask which joint is involved; what seems to trigger your pain; at what time of day the pain is worst; what seems to bring relief, if anything; if there has been redness of the skin at the joint or if it has ever been swollen; if there has been morning stiffness; and for what length of time you've had your symptoms. In addition, your doctor will want to know about what tasks you perform at work every day and what recreational activities you engage in.

A standard physical examination includes inspection of all the joints. It is necessary for the doctor to see which joints are affected, how many are involved, and whether or not the joints on both sides of the body suffer from arthritis.

After a thorough medical history and a complete physical examination, it is possible to make an accurate diagnosis of OA. A "differential diagnosis" (the elimination of all other possible causes of the signs and symptoms that a patient is experiencing) is critical when it comes to making a correct diagnosis of OA because there is no screening test that is recommended by a group such as the American College of Rheumatology or that most physicians can agree is useful. In addition, there are no laboratory tests that can confirm that a patient actually has OA. As a result, eliminating other medical problems is especially important.

To understand this better, let's look at both rheumatoid arthritis (RA) OA. Generally, OA affects only one part of the body in the beginning, such as the left hand and not the right. RA may affect both hands in the early stages. Enlargement of finger joints, redness or a lack of warmth (signs of inflammation), and the absence of such symptoms as fatigue, fever, and weight loss are all characteristic of OA. With OA, urinalysis and blood tests (e.g., complete blood count, blood chemistries, and erythrocyte sedimentation rate) all give results in the normal range. And there is not as much deformity of joints with OA as with RA or gout.

Still, the physician may not be 100 percent certain of the diagnosis. One test can be very helpful in identifying the type of arthritis involved—

examination of the synovial fluid from the affected joint. In addition to helping make a definite diagnosis of the type of arthritis affecting the patient, this test can show whether or not infectious arthritis is present, a condition that is caused by bacteria within the joint space.

Possible Genetic Causes for OA

According to some scientists, inherited genes may be one cause of OA. Although, no specific genetic cause of OA has been determined, recent discoveries have researchers hot on the trail of possible genetic links to OA. In fact, many experts are certain that genetic engineering will play a big role in the future in both the diagnosis and treatment of OA.

While OA is known to run in families, it has not yet been proved to be an inherited condition. One group of researchers compared over 100 sets of identical twins with more than 100 sets of fraternal twins. They found that OA was far more common in both identical twins than in both fraternal twins. Other research has looked at the connections among genes, environment, and the onset of OA. In one report, over 300 families in which OA was present were evaluated. The scientists discovered that the children of these adults with OA had about a 40 percent chance of developing the condition themselves. The researchers hypothesized that a recessive gene was involved in the transmission of OA from one generation to another.

It will undoubtedly be awhile before the genetic component of family clusters of OA is teased out, but a great deal of investigation in this area is under way. One biotechnology company believes it is on the verge of discovering an OA gene and is planning to patent the gene when sufficient data are available.

Unfortunately, the discovery of a gene that causes OA will be significant for only a small segment of the population of those with OA. Joint overuse and injuries will still be the leading culprits in the onset of the disorder. OA will still result from some combination of genes and environment, with the environmental factors playing the bigger role.

Obesity and OA

It should come as no surprise that obesity and the development of OA are linked. The more weight that is placed on weight-bearing joints, the more wear and tear will occur over the years. Every extra pound places increased stress on your joints, especially the knees. But added weight can damage the hips and hands, too. Many researchers have concluded that obesity is one of the leading causes of the high incidence of OA among women. The top cause of OA in men is injury to the knee, but after this form of trauma, obesity is the second leading cause of OA.

Recently the federal government released new guidelines to help individuals determine their body mass index (BMI). This method is an indirect way of measuring obesity, but it can also be used to help determine your risk of developing OA. How do you determine your BMI? It's pretty simple, but you may want to use a calculator. Let's look at a person who is 5 feet, 5 inches tall and weighs 165 pounds.

1. Multiply your weight in pounds by 704 (e.g., 165 × 704).
2. Square your height in inches by multiplying that number by itself (e.g., 65 inches × 65 inches).
3. Divide the result of step 1 by the result of step 2.

The result of the final division gives your BMI. If your BMI is between 25.0 and 29.9, you are considered overweight according to current federal guidelines. If your BMI is over 30, you are considered obese. The only individuals this method does not work for are those who are heavily muscled.

Another way to determine percentage of body fat is to use a type of equipment that emits an electric current that runs through the body. Many health clubs will have this piece of equipment, which really looks like little more than a scale.

Weight loss can help relieve many existing symptoms of OA and people who lose weight can reduce their risk of ever developing OA. Here is an amazing statistic. The incidence of OA of the knee in the American population could be cut by 20 to 30 percent if people lost as little as 11 pounds!

Body weight, however, may be only part of the story. The amount of fat tissue present may play a key role as well. Extra weight can hasten the degeneration of cartilage in the knees and hips. But OA can appear in the hands of overweight individuals, indicating that weight alone is not the cause. According to some researchers, the harmful chemicals that fat cells release into the blood may also cause cartilage degeneration. One study suggests that reduction in body fat, without concurrent loss of weight, resulted in decreased OA symptoms.

There are many options for the treatment of OA, and they will be covered in later chapters.

RHEUMATOID ARTHRITIS (RA)

RA, considered to be an autoimmune disorder, affects only 1 to 2 percent of the population. However, three times as many women suffer from RA as do men. This condition strikes many joints in the body at the same time. In addition, RA causes damage to tissues and organs throughout the body. The onset of RA may occur at any age. However, it most frequently appears in both women and men between the ages of twenty and forty.

The cause of RA remains unknown, but inflammation of the synovial membrane is usually the first sign. The inflammation is thought to be the result of what is called an autoimmune response. In such situations, the body mistakenly identifies a natural part of the body as foreign. Over time, the inflammation leads to overproduction of white blood cells and an over-growth of synovial cells. This, in turn, causes a thickening of the synovial membrane. In a gradual process, the cartilage, bone, ligaments, and tendons are damaged by enzymes and other chemicals released into the body as a result of the autoimmune response.

With the unchecked progression of RA, joint range of motion can be severely impaired due to the excess fibrous tissue the body produces under these conditions. The tissues surrounding the joints are also inflamed, and this further damages the joints.

RA Symptoms

This disorder is characterized by symptoms that are not specific. They are the kinds of symptoms that occur with a number of other medical prob-lems—for example, fatigue, weight loss, loss of appetite, and weakness. People with RA may experience morning stiffness that improves as the day goes on. Strenuous activity can exacerbate the stiffness associated with RA. As the condition worsens, the periods of stiffness lengthen.

The fingers, wrists, knees, ankles, and toes frequently become inflamed because of RA. They become swollen and red and are quite painful. RA usually appears on both sides of the body at the same time (e.g., in the left and right knees). In fact, this symmetrical, bilateral pattern—along with the red, swollen appearance caused by inflammation—is a sign that doctors use to differentiate RA from OA. With RA, the joints at the tips of the fingers are not affected; with OA, they are. RA also affects the tissues; collections of inflammatory cells called rheumatoid nodules form and can be found in tissues throughout the body. It is estimated that 20 percent of patients develop rheumatoid nodules. Over time, RA progresses and joints become deformed. This can occur in months or over many years. The person's range of motion in the affected area can become severely limited.

Other symptoms of RA include muscle atrophy and even atrophy of the skin around the affected joints. There may be dryness of the mouth, eyes, and other mucous membranes. Some individuals may develop carpal tunnel syndrome. Unfortunately, RA can at times lead to pericarditis, inflammation of the membrane that covers the heart. The membrane covering the lungs may become inflamed as well. In some people with RA, the spleen becomes enlarged. And there may also be blindness due to serious inflammation of the outer layers of the eyes.

Diagnosing RA

It is not easy to diagnose this condition. Usually, the symptoms need to be present for many weeks before a doctor can confidently diagnose RA. As with OA, the initial diagnosis is made by ruling out the existence of other conditions that can cause the same physical symptoms. Again, as with OA, the physician or other health care provider will take a complete medical history and perform a thorough physical examination. If a doctor discovers that multiple, symmetrical joints on both sides of the body are red, swollen, and warm to the touch, this will strongly indicate the presence of RA.

What complicates the diagnosis of this disorder is the fact that it can be made only when the symptoms are present. And the symptoms of RA do go into remission at times. It is also a challenge to diagnose RA in joints that are deep in the body, such as the hips. However, the diagnosis of RA can be confirmed through the use of X rays and a number of different laboratory tests.

During the medical history, honesty on the part of the patient is essential to an accurate diagnosis. Many people try to minimize the pain they feel or underestimate the impact the disease has had on the range of motion of their joints. Some people are reluctant to acknowledge how fatigued they have become, how severely they feel their disability, and how greatly it affects their daily life.

As important as it is to answer truthfully the questions the doctor asks, it is just as important to tell the health care provider about symptoms and pain that are not asked about. Men, more than women, tend to minimize the pain and discomfort they are experiencing and to be more reluctant to discuss issues with their doctors and other health care providers.

The information that a patient provides a physician is critical in determining the course of treatment for RA, or for any other disorder. Being stoical or putting on a brave face can hinder the effectiveness of treatment or possibly even lead to the wrong approach to managing RA symptoms.

After different laboratory tests are performed, a doctor can be more certain if the patient's physical symptoms are caused by RA. The first useful step is to examine the synovial fluid. This is done by taking a small sample of this fluid from the affected joint and finding out how many white blood cells are present. These cells help the body fight off infection, but they are also involved in the body's anti-inflammatory response. If the existence of synovitis—inflammation of the synovial membrane—is demonstrated by this test, a physician can be much more certain that the diagnosis of RA is correct.

If a patient has had active symptoms for six months or more, and the suspicion of RA is high, the existence of this disorder can be confirmed by the use of X rays. In the later stages of RA, but not in the early stages, the X rays will show such characteristics of active RA as bony erosions of the affected joint and narrowing of the joint space. The presence of these phenomena strongly indicates that the patient is suffering from RA.

There is another lab test that can be quite useful when making a diagnosis of RA. This test checks for the presence in the body of an abnormal protein called the rheumatoid factor. Approximately 85 percent of patients with RA have this abnormal protein present in their blood. The more severe the RA, the greater the amount of this protein will be found in the patient's blood. Some patients may not have this protein in their blood sample in the early stages of the disease, but it will show up as the disease progresses.

As good as the test for rheumatoid factor is, it is not always definitive. The abnormal protein involved can also be found in the blood of people who are suffering from a range of different disorders. In addition, people with autoimmune disorders other than RA may also have this protein in their blood. But in conjunction with a good differential diagnosis and other tests, the lab exam for the rheumatoid factor can be quite valuable.

How do people with RA fare? It seems that approximately 10 percent of patients who are diagnosed with RA experience a complete remission within one year of diagnosis. And 40 to 65 percent of patients find that the disease goes into remission within two years. In both of these groups, rheumatoid factor levels are low and the symptoms that are experienced are usually relatively mild. That's the good news. The bad news is that if RA persists for more than two years, the situation is quite different and the prognosis is not good. For people with RA for longer than two years, there is a much higher incidence of deformity of the affected joints. Unfortunately, people who suffer from RA long term also have a lower overall survival rate because the disease can affect the heart, lungs, eyes, and intestines, causing serious damage.

Just as those who are significantly overweight or obese are at higher risk of RA, smokers may find that their habit increases their risk of developing this condition. A study published in the *Journal of Rheumatology* in March 1999 suggests that the risk of developing RA may be increased by as much as 50 percent among those who smoke either cigarettes or cigars. The researchers looked at 361 patients with RA and compared them to nearly 6,000 randomly chosen individuals. The authors concluded that smoking as little as once a day appeared to significantly increase the risk for men and women in the development of RA.

Although the link between smoking and RA has not been firmly established, as it has been between smoking and cancer, it is an area of research that should concern those with RA, at risk of developing the condition, and all smokers as well. Many smokers are aware of the smoking–cancer connection, but one recent study in the *Journal of the American Medical Association* has shown that approximately 66 percent of smokers are unaware that smoking is linked with many serious illnesses other than cancer.

"LEAKY GUT" SYNDROME AND FOOD ALLERGIES

"Leaky gut" syndrome is associated with RA in some instances. Holistic practitioners use the term *dysbiosis* to describe circumstances under which the intestine is not functioning properly. The gut has two main functions: to admit what the body needs and to keep out what it does not need. When the intestine is disordered, the capacity for the assimilation and absorption of food is decreased. In addition, the gut is less able to serve as an effective barrier. If the intestinal lining is raw and inflamed, proteins and other molecules that are not fully digested are able to pass through, and the body targets them as foreign. The immune system goes into action and creates antibodies to fight the "invaders." This immune response results in the development of a food allergy. This reaction may be immediate or it may be delayed. (There are recommendations for treating dysbiosis in chapter 7.)

GOUT AND PSEUDOGOUT

Gout

Today gout is often linked with men who overindulge in alcohol or with individuals consuming large quantities of red meat. In the past, gout was known as a rich man's disease because it seemed to be connected with the cuisine and lifestyle of the upper classes. However, medical science has taught us that gout is a systemic disease. Its main characteristic is increased blood levels of uric acid, with an increase in uric acid production greater than excretion. It is the high levels of uric acid that cause the repeated attacks of acute arthritis known as gout.

In the beginning, gout is usually confined to a single joint. Over time, chronic arthritis may develop, affecting and deforming many joints in the body. Gout occurs more frequently in men than in women and usually begins after the age of thirty. It is generally not until after menopause that women begin to develop gout. As with other arthritic conditions, obesity can increase the risk of gout for both men and women. Research shows that nearly 50 percent of those with gout are at least 15 percent above their recommended weight.

There are two types of gout—inherited, or primary, gout and secondary gout. Sometimes both conditions exist at the same time. With primary gout, an increase in the production of uric acid by the body leads to elevated levels of uric acid in the blood. There may also be a reduced excretion of uric acid in the urine. With secondary gout, high blood levels of uric acid may be caused by a wide range of factors. Chronic kidney failure can cause gout, as can the use of diuretics. Cancer chemotherapy, with the rapid destruction of cells in the body, can lead to the production of the chemical precursors of uric acid and this can cause gout. In addition, gout is associated with such disorders as leukemia, multiple myeloma, and psoriasis.

An acute attack of gout begins when sodium urate crystals are formed in the body and deposited into a joint and the surrounding synovial membrane. The body responds to this by sending white blood cells to the area as part of its immune response. The white blood cells overrun the crystals. However, as they do, they release a number of chemical substances that cause inflammation. This produces the acute arthritic attack.

These urate crystals can also cause problems in other parts of the body, such as the subcutaneous tissue, bones, tendons, and kidneys. When urate crystals accumulate, they create lesions. The lesions are called *tophi*. Tophi are urate crystals surrounded by cells that the body sends to fight off the "foreign invader" that is causing it harm. When tophi form within and around the joint, they can do great damage, leading to chronic gouty arthritis. Chronic gout can be exacerbated by the presence of OA.

Although a majority of people with high blood levels of uric acid develop gout, many do not. Paradoxically, both a rapid rise in blood uric acid levels and a rapid fall in these levels can bring on an attack of gout. In addition, excessive excretion of uric acid in the urine can lead to the development of painful kidney stones, possibly serious kidney damage, and even kidney failure.

Pseudogout

The accumulation in the body of crystals of calcium pyrophosphate within a joint leads to the onset of pseudogout. This disease almost always occurs in people over the age of sixty and its symptoms are confined to the joints. People with pseudogout usually have normal blood uric acid levels. Frequently, it takes the examination of X rays—which show calcification of the cartilage of affected joints—to reveal the presence of this disorder. The examination of fluid from the affected joint can show the presence of calcium pyrophosphate crystals and confirm the diagnosis of pseudogout that was suggested by the X rays.

Pseudogout may lead to attacks of chronic arthritis in the knees, wrists, and other large joints. This condition is associated with other medical problems, such as diabetes, excessive iron in the tissues, hyperthyroidism, and hyperparathyroidism.

Gout Symptoms

Gout occurs without warning, frequently at night. The most common site for an attack is the big toe, affecting 75 percent of those who suffer from gout attacks at some time. Gout can afflict the knees, ankles, and feet, often with several sites being affected simultaneously. Common symptoms include swelling, tenderness of the affected area, redness and warmth of the skin over the joint, slight to moderate fever, and gradually increasing pain in the joint.

Attacks of gout may occur months or even years apart. However, over time, the intervals between the attacks usually become shorter. If a person starts to experience gout attacks before the age of fifty, the disease may progress quite rapidly. Gout is associated with high blood pressure, kidney disease, diabetes, artherosclerosis, and uric acid kidney stones.

A doctor can make a diagnosis of gout based on the appearance of the joint and the typical symptoms that the patient reports. Blood tests can be used to confirm the physician's suspicions. Examination of fluid from the affected joint will show high levels of urate crystals and X rays will also provide information to confirm the diagnosis.

FIBROMYALGIA SYNDROME

What does the word *fibromyalgia* mean? *Fibro* indicates that the fibrous ligaments and tendons of the body are involved in the condition. *My* stands for muscles. And *algia* means that it causes pain. So the word *fibromyalgia* describes a condition that causes pain in the tendons, ligaments, and muscles. What is a syndrome? It is a set of symptoms that, in combination with physical findings, define a particular condition.

It may come as a surprise to many people, but some experts think that, next to OA, fibromyalgia syndrome is the most common rheumatic condition. Approximately 20 percent of all visits to a rheumatologist involve fibromyalgia. It is estimated that 3.7 million Americans suffer from this syndrome. Nearly 90 percent of all patients with symptoms of this syndrome are female. Although the onset of fibromyalgia may occur as early as age twenty, it can arise at any time in individuals between twenty and sixty years of age. It is frequently found among older women.

The pain caused by fibromyalgia is diffuse. Most people experience it as an achiness and stiffness all over the body, but it is more relegated to muscular tissue. With fibromyalgia, muscle tissue can be very painful to touch. Those suffering from this disorder do have areas of the body that are particularly sensitive to pain. However, they are often unaware of these "trigger points" until pressure is applied to them.

Fibromyalgia is also associated with chronic fatigue. In fact, some experts believe that fibromyalgia is simply a metabolic stepping-stone to chronic fatigue syndrome. It is quite common for people afflicted with this condition to feel tired and worn out all day. Many people awaken feeling unrested even though they have slept throughout the night. Although the individual did sleep, the fibromyalgia probably caused sleep disturbances that account for the weariness on waking and throughout the day. One way to describe the feeling is to imagine working out all day in intense training. The soreness and aching you would feel would be due to high levels of lactic acid buildup in muscle tissue. Fibromyalgia patients feel like this without moving a muscle!

Fibromyalgia is difficult to diagnose, in large part because at present it is so poorly understood. It is quite common for the disorder to disrupt a person's life for years before it is correctly diagnosed. It is only over the past several years that physicians are becoming aware that fibromyalgia syndrome is a distinct clinical entity.

Interestingly, unlike other related conditions, fibromyalgia does not cause inflammation. Neither does it do any damage to the joints, muscles, or connective tissues. In fact, the absence of inflammation is a key characteristic that helps differentiate fibromyalgia from RA. Unlike OA and RA, fibromyalgia does not result in the deformity of joints. However, the pain and fatigue associated with this condition can be intense at times.

Clinicians working with fibromyalgia have seen that there are diverse factors that contribute to the problem, and although the cause of this condition has not yet been determined, there are several theories as to its origin. Some experts think that the condition may begin after a severe bout of the flu or another traumatic illness. Other researchers suspect that this disorder may be linked to extreme emotional or physical distress. And still others believe that microtrauma to the muscles is involved in the onset of fibromyalgia. It is hypothesized that these traumas cause a decrease in blood flow to the muscles. As a result of the decreased flow of blood, the individual feels weak and fatigued.

There are also experts who think that the sleep disturbance that seems to be caused by fibromyalgia is actually the underlying cause of the disorder. Studies have demonstrated that people with fibromyalgia do not benefit from the restorative stage of deep sleep (i.e., delta-wave sleep). In one experiment, healthy volunteers had their sleep interrupted so that they did not experience deep delta-wave sleep. These experimental subjects developed the symptoms that are characteristic of fibromyalgia syndrome.

Among the other suggested causes of fibromyalgia are central nervous system abnormalities, disturbances in the production of serotonin or in serotonin metabolism, low blood pressure, and low levels of somatomedin C.

Still other theories of causes include immune response abnormalities in the intestines to various foods, dysbiosis (abnormal flora in the gut), adrenal exhaustion caused by long-term stress, hypothyroidism, and a reduced ability for muscle cells to process lactic acid.

The truth is that probably several of these factors are present in the individual at the same time. Reducing the pain associated with fibromyalgia can go a long way in supporting a total wellness plan for coping with this condition.

Fibromyalgia Symptoms

The primary symptom is pain. To describe it, people frequently use the words "burning" and "gnawing." Usually the pain begins in one part of the body and is localized there. However, over time, it spreads to other areas. For example, pain may begin in the neck, but spread to the lower back or the leg muscles. Often people with fibromyalgia complain of symptoms that are commonly associated with the flu. The stiffness and aches and pains are worse in the morning for most people. But some level of pain is generally present throughout the day. Pain may increase with exercise. Other factors that intensify fibromyalgia pain include wet, hot, cold, or damp weather; emotional stress; sleep disturbances; and physical stress.

People with this syndrome frequently complain that they no longer have the energy to engage in the activities they used to enjoy, such as exercising and walking. Moderate to severe fatigue is common, as are sensations of numbness and tingling. Many people feel a swelling of the hands.

Those who suffer from fibromyalgia are also more likely to suffer from a wide range of other signs and symptoms of illness. For example, people with fibromyalgia are more likely than others to suffer from migraines or tension headaches. And many of those who suffer from this syndrome are allergic to a host of medications as well as to large numbers of the chemicals that have been put into our environment, which is increasingly flooded with synthetic substances.

Fibromyalgia is also associated with depression. Approximately 25 percent of people with this syndrome are clinically depressed at any given time, and many of these people have histories of depression. Nearly 50 percent of those who suffer from fibromyalgia experience an episode of depression at some point in their lives. This figure is much higher than that for the general population. As is the case with the link between fibromyalgia and sleep disturbances, it is not clear whether the depression is a result of the fibromyalgia or is itself a cause of the syndrome. In addition, chronic long-term pain on its own can cause depression. There is a body of evidence suggesting some correlation among the mechanisms that cause both depression and fibromyalgia.

Although those suffering from fibromyalgia have a higher incidence of depression than does the general population, their rates of depression are comparable to those who suffer from other health problems such as irritable bowel syndrome, restless leg syndrome, and anxiety. Of those suffering from fibromyalgia, 33 percent experience irritable bowel syndrome, 50 percent suffer from anxiety, and 75 percent experience restless leg syndrome.

Diagnosing Fibromyalgia Syndrome

There are no physical, objective changes in a person that a physician can use to diagnose this condition. OA and RA are relatively easy to diagnose in comparison with fibromyalgia. Blood tests, tissue biopsies, and X rays of these patients usually all come back normal. For many years physicians believed that the syndrome was of purely psychological origin. There may be those who still believe so. However, despite the lack of evidence from either lab tests or physical examination, it is now believed that this is a true physical condition. An increasing number of doctors know this and are better able to recognize the syndrome.

The American College of Rheumatology (ACR) in 1990 set forth a set of criteria in 1990 that can be used to diagnose fibromyalgia. The patient must experience pain for at least three months. This pain must be felt on both sides of the body as well as above and below the waist. The ACR also identified eighteen pain trigger points. Physicians use a device called a dolorimeter to apply nine pounds of pressure to these trigger points. There must be pain at eleven of these points to indicate fibromyalgia. When this procedure is performed, the patient will feel significant pain, enough to flinch or make a sound. Recent research has led clinicians to include patients' reports of poor quality of sleep and fatigue, along with the ACR criteria, as indications of fibromyalgia.

Several lab tests may be needed to diagnose this syndrome. Blood tests may be done so the doctor can rule out lupus, Lyme disease, RA, hypothyroidism, and other conditions with similar symptoms. Diagnosing this syndrome involves more than eliminating the possibility of other conditions with similar symptomatology. The syndrome can be present alongside other medical problems. Studies suggest that one out of ten patients with RA also suffers from fibromyalgia syndrome. It is vital that anyone who feels that he or she may be suffering from fibromyalgia see a doctor who is experienced with the syndrome. A rheumatologist may be the best choice because other physicians may not be aware of the ACR criteria or not apply the correct amount of pressure to the eighteen trigger points, leading to a misdiagnosis of the problem.

BURSITIS

There are about 150 small fluid-filled sacs that act as cushions in the parts of the body where muscles or tendons move over bones or muscles. These sacs are called bursas. These structures prevent direct contact between the bones and muscles or tendons. By so doing, they prevent the development of problems that are caused by friction among these parts of the body.

Sometimes the bursas can become inflamed. As a result, a person feels pain and experiences swelling at the site of the problem. This inflammation is referred to as bursitis. The bursas that are most commonly affected are at the hips, knees, feet, shoulders, and elbows. Bursitis may appear at times to be indistinguishable from arthritis, as it produces similar symptoms. However, a major difference between the two conditions is that bursitis does not affect the joint itself, as arthritis does. Instead, bursitis affects the tissues surrounding the joint. In general, bursitis will usually clear up on its own within a few weeks. It can become a chronic problem if the patient does not take measures to prevent its recurrence.

The most common cause of bursitis is repetitive motion. The stress from such an action causes inflammation. So-called "tennis elbow" is a good example of this. Also, bursitis of the shoulder can result from placing too great a strain on the area, as with serving in tennis. The pressure from a blow, a fall, or a bump can also cause bursitis. Something as simple as frequently resting an elbow on a hard desk for a long period of time (e.g., at work) can also lead to the inflammation known as bursitis.

For some people, the bursas of the hips can become inflamed when problems with the feet cause them to favor one foot or the other. This upsets the proper alignment of the legs and puts strain on the hips, causing bursitis. This can occur from something as common as wearing shoes with worn-out heels. Bunions are actually a form of bursitis, usually located near the big toe, which can be caused by shoes that do not fit properly.

Bursitis is quite common among people with arthritis because many of them develop poor body mechanics as they try, ineffectively, to cope with the chronic pain they feel and the lack of range of motion that comes with this disorder. In so doing, the simple activities of daily life, performed incorrectly, lead to bursitis.

Pain is the number one symptom of this problem. It is usually dull but persistent. It can interfere with getting a good night's sleep. Movement frequently increases the pain. Although the pain is generally localized to the area around the inflamed bursas, it may spread or radiate along an arm or leg. The bursas are tender when touched.

Diagnosing Bursitis

The primary method of diagnosing this problem is physical inspection of the joints and the surrounding tissue. Although bursitis itself does not show up on X rays, sometimes one will be taken to make sure that there is not some other cause for the problem. The patient will be asked a few simple questions by the physician to aid in making a diagnosis. The patient will likely be asked how long he or she has experienced the pain, if it has occurred before, if it is related to any injury or activity, what makes it worse, and if the patient has taken any medications in the past for this or similar pain.

When a diagnosis is made, there are simple treatments available, although preventing it from occurring in the first place, if possible, is always wise.

Preventing Bursitis

- Keep muscles well conditioned.
- Avoid prolonged repetitive activity.
- Develop good posture.
- Warm up properly before exercising.
- Stretch your muscles to maintain flexibility.
- Strengthen your muscles with regular physical activity.
- Use protective gear during sports activities.
- Wear adequate shoes and athletic shoes.
- Use a seat cushion and lumbar pillow when making long drives.
- Avoid leaning on your elbows.
- Get up from your desk every thirty minutes.
- At the computer, keep your eyes level with the top of the screen and sit up straight.

CHRONIC FATIGUE SYNDROME

Chronic fatigue syndrome (CFS) was first recognized in 1988 and is marked by severe and debilitating fatigue. It can last for more than six months. CFS is not fully understood today and remains a great puzzle. Although CFS and fibromyalgia are considered to be distinct entities, there are some researchers who are beginning to suspect that they may actually be caused by the same mechanism or may even be the same disease.

According to the Centers for Disease Control and Prevention, anywhere from 4 to 10 out of every 100,000 adults is affected by CFS at some time in their lives. Four times as many women as men are diagnosed with CFS, usually between the ages of twenty-five and forty-five.

As understanding of CFS has increased, there are those who suspect that it may affect many more people than previously thought. However, too many unknowns remain. For example, it is not understood what brings on the disorder or how to treat it. There are even scientists who believe that there is no such disease as CFS, that it is really a collection of symptoms caused by other undiagnosed problems.

For a diagnosis of CFS, persistent severe fatigue and at least four of the following symptoms must be present: impaired concentration or short-term memory, disturbed sleep, muscle pain, fatigue that lasts for more than twenty-four hours after exertion, sore throat, tender lymph nodes, multiple joint pain without redness or swelling, and new headaches.

Because CFS is so prevalent and affects so many people, quite a bit of research into this condition is now under way. Investigators are looking at a wide range of factors that may be involved. Some view CFS as a multiple metabolic syndrome in which a variety of long-term factors play key roles. Such factors include stress, exposure to environmental toxins (e.g., mercury, lead, pesticides), poor nutrition and resultant vitamin and mineral deficiency, and excessive use of drugs (e.g., antibiotics). Researchers are also studying the possible association of CFS with hyperinsulinemia and hypothyroidism.

4
Cox-2 Inhibitors: A Revolution in the Treatment of Inflammation

The term *Cox-2 inhibitors* describes compounds—both the natural versions and the synthetic—that inhibit an enzyme in the body called cyclooxygenase-2. Pharmaceutical firms have created two popular prescription versions of these drugs—Celebrex and Vioxx. These Cox-2 inhibitors are fast becoming two of the most prescribed pharmaceutical drugs on the market, with recent reports that one of them has surpassed the anti-impotence medication Viagra as the fastest-selling prescription drug in history. Nearly seven million prescriptions for Celebrex were filled during its first six months on the market, compared with about 5.3 million for Viagra (IMS Health, 1999). Sales of Celebrex in the first six months added up to about $600 million, compared with Viagra's $552 million in sales its first six months beginning in April 1998. Celebrex and Vioxx were two of the top twenty most prescribed drugs in 2000 (*Drug Topics*, April 16, 2001). Also, pain relievers (including the nonsteroidal anti-inflammatory [NSAID] over-the-counter medications) are consistently top sellers in the multibillion-dollar over-the-counter drug market. You will see their ads on TV, on the Internet, in newspapers and magazines, and hear them on the radio. Interestingly, modern scientists for the pharmaceutical companies were not the first to discover Cox-2 inhibitors. Healers since the time of Hippocrates have known about the extraordinary healing powers of plants with natural Cox-2 inhibiting ability.

The new approach toward integrative care can only benefit the public and health care professionals alike. The Cox-2 inhibitors, whether in the form of synthetic drugs or natural herbs, can help patients and their health care providers deal with the inflammation that results from any number of "bodymind" disorders that afflict people at present. In fact, incorporating natural versions of Cox-2 inhibitors into health care will probably always be helpful to patients. It seems that the Cox-2 inflammation process may be involved in the onset of many diseases. Thus, long before symptoms appear, the living bodymind may be struggling with, and may eventually succumb to, inflammation caused by these potent enzymes.

The whole story is yet to be told about the synthetic Cox-2 inhibitors, but the promise of time-tested natural remedies that inhibit Cox-2 inflammation may turn out to be a major advance in medical care. Only time will validate the synthetic inhibitors' safety. Western science is now able to identify the chemical constituents of many herbs that inhibit Cox-2-induced inflammation. With this form of treatment, relief through symptom suppression may not be the whole story. With Cox-2 inhibitors, it may even be possible for the disease process to be slowed, which can aid the body in achieving a balance of health once again.

Whom can Cox-2 inhibitors potentially help? As discussed, those with chronic and acute inflammation may benefit. Apparently, people with colon cancer, breast cancer, esophageal cancer, bladder cancer, and skin cancer may benefit. And there may be a role for Cox-2 inhibitors in the management of Alzheimer's disease. (See chapter 5 for more information on the Cox-2 connection in Alzheimer's and cancer.) For the purposes of this chapter, we will focus on another important group of people for whom these chemicals may be lifesavers—those with inflammatory disorders.

COX-2 INHIBITORS: THE STORY SO FAR

Celebrex (celecoxib) and Vioxx (rofecoxib) are the most well-known Cox-2 inhibitors on the market. They are targeted at treating arthritis and other forms of inflammation, and it is claimed that they can treat arthritis with a lower risk of causing bleeding or stomach ulcers than comes with either aspirin or NSAIDs.

Celebrex was approved in late 1998 and Vioxx's approval followed shortly afterward in 1999. Celebrex was the first prescription drug to reach $1 billion in sales in the United States in its first year on the market. Its worldwide sales reached $3 billion in the year 2000. Although they were introduced only two years ago, these two Cox-2 inhibitors account for about 40 percent of all drugs purchased to treat arthritis and for 60 percent of all dollars spent on these products. They cost about ten times more than older anti-inflammatory drugs. For example, treating arthritis with an over-the-counter version of aspirin or ibuprofen would cost about fifty cents a day, as compared with three to six dollars a day for Cox-2 inhibitors.

Many advertising dollars have gone into promoting these new agents; Vioxx was the most heavily advertised drug on TV in the year 2000. In one survey, 90 percent of Americans said they saw drug ads on TV and 40 percent said they talked to their doctors about taking the drugs they saw advertised.

NSAIDs have been on the market and in use for decades. They act by inhibiting two enzymes, Cox-1 and Cox-2. Two examples of NSAIDs are ibuprofen and naproxen. Cox-1, "the good Cox," is a chemical that plays a role in the production of the chemical mediators—prostaglandins—that help protect the stomach against ulcers. Cox-2 is an enzyme that produces prostaglandins which cause inflammation.

The new drugs—Cox-2 inhibitors—represent an advance over the NSAIDs because they inhibit only Cox-2, which causes inflammation. They do not have an impact on Cox-1, which has a beneficial effect on the body. Because they do not inhibit Cox-1, these new drugs are expected to be able to treat pain and inflammation without causing any of the serious gastrointestinal side effects that are associated with the use of aspirin and the many popular NSAIDs available today.

The medical industry was extremely excited when the FDA approved celecoxib (Celebrex) in 1998. It seemed that, finally, there was a drug available to treat inflammation as effectively as the existing NSAIDs without the serious side effects. In its first ninety days on the market, 2.5 million prescriptions were written for Celebrex. (But the big new drug story that captured the public's attention at that time involved another billion-dollar blockbuster product called sildenafil—or Viagra.) But Cox-2 inhibitors are still not without controversy.

COMPARING RISKS

NSAIDs are used widely in the United States. Over 70 million prescriptions are written for these drugs each year and more than 30 *billion* pills are sold over the counter annually. Although the risks associated with NSAIDs may not be significantly greater than those for other synthetic drugs that are on the market, with so many people now taking the drugs, awareness of potential side effects is important.

Some data suggest that Cox-2 inhibitors may not be as free from potential side effects as originally thought, but for now they appear to have significant benefits over the other NSAIDs. NSAID therapy can not only be harsh on the gastrointestinal tract (causing gastric ulceration) but may also be damaging to the liver and kidneys. It is estimated that 25 percent of patients using NSAIDs experience some kind of side effect, and about 5 percent develop a serious health consequence (e.g., massive GI bleed, acute renal failure). Cox-2 inhibitors were developed in order to bypass these potential side effects. As stated earlier, they work by inhibiting the "bad" Cox-2 enzyme while sparing the "good" Cox-1 enzyme, which has a protective role in maintaining the integrity of the gastroduodenal mucosa.[1] How serious are the health problems associated with NSAIDs? Problems range from mild stomach upset to peptic ulcers and kidney or liver failure. Adverse effects of NSAIDs, which are mainly related to gastrointestinal bleeding, can be serious, and throughout the world cause about 260,000 hospitalizations and 26,000 deaths a year. But remember, each day at least 30 million people take NSAIDs.[2] There are a number of ways to lower the severity or risk of side effects from NSAIDs, and these will be discussed later in the book.

Introduced about 100 years ago, aspirin was the first successful analgesic or pain reliever. It was synthesized based on a chemical constituent found in the bark of the white willow tree *(Salix alba)*. Acetaminophen was brought to the market about fifty years ago and the NSAIDs made their debut about a quarter of a century ago. Each type of analgesic has a certain level of effectiveness, and each can produce unwanted side effects, mostly gastrointestinal. And each product has been advertised as surpassing the previous drug in effectiveness and with fewer adverse effects.

Today the Cox-2 inhibitors are sometimes referred to as "super aspirin." The new drugs were shown in clinical trials to be as effective as aspirin in relieving the pain of arthritis, but without the associated side effects. In fact, the Cox-2 inhibitors produced no more side effects than did the placebos used in the trials. Some clinicians believe that Cox-2 inhibitors may be of particular benefit to older individuals, especially those with a history of ulcers, and to people who are taking steroids. The reasons for this will be discussed in later chapters.

However, data are beginning to appear that suggest that Cox-2 inhibitors may not be as free from potential side effects as originally thought. Recently published literature challenges the notion that Cox-2 inhibitors won't harm the gastrointestinal tract.[3] This research has reported the inhibition of the Cox-1 and Cox-2 enzymes by the body and that Cox-2 also has potential to affect the gut. Further research also suggests that when cyclooxygenase (Cox-1 or Cox-2) is inhibited, a different inflammatory product (termed lipoxygenase, or LOX) is increased. LOX-induced leukotrienes (inflammatory mediators) are as dangerous to brain cells as Cox-induced prostaglandins in that they also may cause inflammation and potentially diseases associated with inflammation, such as cancer, Alzheimer's, and arthritis.

Another problem exists with Cox-2 inhibitors and their effects on angiogenesis (the formation of new blood vessels), as described in chapter 5. Cox-2 inhibitors block the Cox-2 enzyme and subsequently interfere with the growth and initiation of these new vessels. The more blood vessels formed in and around a tumor, the more food can get to the cancer and allow it to grow and spread. Although the inhibition of angiogenesis may be beneficial in reducing tumor growth, new blood vessels are imperative to wound and ulcer healing. These data raise questions concerning whether selective Cox-2 drugs are safer for the gastrointestinal tract than older NSAIDS after all, because inhibiting angiogenesis may result in ulcer complications. Unfortunately, the Cox-2 inhibitors may still retain some of the side effects seen with traditional NSAIDs—namely, effects on the kidney that may indirectly cause an increase in blood pressure and the incidence of hypertension, swelling, and other cardiovascular problems.[4]

At present, according to the best information available, Cox-2 inhibitors have great potential in the war against inflammation. However, there may be still unidentified risks involved with the widespread use of these pharmaceutical drugs, as with any medicine taken by so many people. Some individuals may not wish to take the pharmaceutical drugs for various reasons. Some individuals may be elderly; some may have a disease such as cardiovascular disease, which complicates drug therapy many times; and others may just not want to take pharmaceutical drugs as the initial agent used for a particular problem. Whatever the case, it's important to realize that there are options for you when health care becomes an issue—choices in the kinds of medications you put in your body and the quality of health care you seek.

More and more, trained and qualified health care professionals—physicians, pharmacists, nurses, and the like—are becoming knowledgeable in the field of natural medicine. Ask them for advice on issues pertaining to your health, and always tell your physician and pharmacist what dietary supplements you are taking along with the prescribed drugs. There may be important interactions between the medicines that you and your doctor need to be aware of.

5

The Cox-2 Connection in Alzheimer's and Cancer

As the Cox-2 inhibitors are working their "magic" in the realm of arthritis and inflammation, some exciting news about other uses for these drugs has recently surfaced. The pro-inflammatory Cox-2 enzyme is also produced in human colon cancer cells, and NSAIDs (nonsteroidal anti-inflammatory drugs) are thought to delay the progress of colon tumors possibly by causing apoptosis (programmed cell death) of the tumor cells.[1,2] With interest from the public in taking proactive steps to reducing risks associated with cancer, Cox-2-inhibiting compounds could provide a promising role in an overall prevention plan.

The risk of developing Alzheimer's disease, which is thought to involve an inflammatory component, may also be reduced by chronic use of NSAIDs.[3] Statistics show that there are over 4 million people afflicted with Alzheimer's disease in the United States, costing our health care system more than $100 billion annually (Alzheimer's Association, 2001). The U.S. federal government estimates that expenditures for Alzheimer's research topped $466 million in 2000.

Alternative therapies for these diseases add weapons for the health care professional and the patient in the war waged against these diseases. In this chapter, the connection between Alzheimer's and Cox-2 inhibition and between cancer and Cox-2 inhibition, along with alternative treatments, is covered.

Note that for discussion purposes in this chapter, NSAIDs generally are considered to be both Cox-1 and Cox-2 inhibitors. Because NSAIDs can also inhibit Cox-1, they can damage the lining of the stomach. They have been reported to cause stomach bleeding and ulcers, potential kidney and liver damage, and over 26,000 deaths each year. Cox-2 inhibitors are not reported to damage the intestinal lining to any appreciable extent, yet new research may hold a different outcome.

COX-2 INHIBITION AND ALZHEIMER'S DISEASE—THE SCIENCE

Alzheimer's disease is named after the scientist Alois Alzheimer, who first identified it in 1907. This neurodegenerative disease causes selective neuronal loss in brain regions involved in memory, language, personality, and cognition. Age is the major risk factor for development of Alzheimer's disease. Onset is uncommon before sixty years of age, but early onset occurs in 5 to 10 percent of patients, possibly due to an inherited mutation in one of several genes. The incidence of Alzheimer's increases with age, doubling every five years between ages sixty and eighty-five. Some evidence suggests that the incidence of the disease may decline at advanced ages over eighty-five. The disease occurs more often in women than in men, but it is debated whether this prevalence is because susceptibility is greater in women or simply because women live longer. Limited education and a history of head trauma may also be factors in development of the disease. Some things to look for in diagnosing Alzheimer's include:

- Dementia established by clinical examination from a qualified physician
- Deficits in two or more areas of cognition (i.e., language, memory, perception)
- Progressive worsening of memory and other cognitive function; as the disease progresses, patient experiences impairment in activities of daily living and altered behavioral patterns
- No disturbance of consciousness
- Onset between ages forty and ninety, but most often after age sixty-five
- Absence of other diseases and/or drug use that may account for deficits in memory and cognition

While scientists don't know for sure what causes Alzheimer's disease, progress is being made in its research. Many scientists now believe that inflammation may be an important component of the Alzheimer's disease process. Examination of the brain in deceased Alzheimer's patients shows inflammatory changes in addition to the classic features, such as the plaques. It is unknown if the inflammatory changes are the primary causes of or a response to neuronal degeneration. The amyloid and protein plaques found in Alzheimer's patients' brains, which are hallmarks of the disease, may point to an inflammatory response. These "tangles" provoke an immune reaction that creates oxidative stress, causing free radical damage and tissue destruction that result in a loss of blood supply to the brain. Researchers believe that NSAIDs may influence inflammation by interfering with the actions of some of these "folded" proteins, with the possible result of enhanced cognitive performance, delayed onset of the disease, and suppressed inflammation in the Alzheimer's-afflicted brain. [4,5]

ANTI-INFLAMMATORY DRUGS AND ALZHEIMER'S

Although the mechanism by which NSAIDs inhibit development of Alzheimer's disease is unproved, a common feature of NSAIDs is their ability to inhibit the cyclooxygenase enzymes Cox-1 and Cox-2. It is thought that Cox-1 mediates the major side effects of NSAIDs, while Cox-2 is involved in inflammation. NSAIDs block a protein known as nuclear factor kappa B (NFkB), which promotes the production of three cytokines elevated in Alzheimer's disease: tumor necrosis factor (TNF), interleukin-1 (IL-1), and interleukin-6 (IL-6). Cytokines are produced by immune cells and cause immune cells to multiply and create oxidative chemicals, such as hydrogen peroxide, that generate free radicals. The free radicals, in turn, drive the production of more inflammatory cytokines and more activation. All three inflammatory mediators increase naturally with a person's age, but in Alzheimer's patients, levels are highly elevated. These three provoke a host of destructive immune responses, such as the complement pathway, which involves a protein that may eventually destroy host cells. By blocking NFkB, ibuprofen reduces inflammatory or "bad" cytokine levels, stops the production of free radicals, and deactivates immune cells. Thus, NSAIDs decrease cytokine production and, in turn, inflammation.

The second way NSAIDs work is by interfering with an enzyme that provokes pro-inflammatory substances known as prostaglandins, which are created from arachidonic acid, an omega-6 fatty acid found in cell membranes. There are several types of prostaglandins. One type maintains the lining of the stomach and promotes kidney function, initiated by Cox-1.

Another is a type that generates free radicals, initiated by Cox-2. By blocking prostaglandins, Cox inhibitors lessen the free radical attack on brain tissue. Free radicals not only damage tissue directly, but they also provoke the production of glutamate and nitric oxide, which can be damaging as well. Plus, free radicals can also activate NFkB, setting off a new round of cytokines and free radical production. Free radicals may damage blood vessels, causing an increase in cardiovascular diseases such as atherosclerosis (hardening of the arteries).

CURRENT RESEARCH ON ALZHEIMER'S

Whether or not NSAIDs can reduce the number of senile plaques and neurofibrillary tangles is still under investigation. These abnormal clumps are made up of pieces of proteins known as amyloid peptides. A study published in 1996 reported that in cell cultures, the steroidal drug dexamethasone decreased the amount of amyloid plaques by 66 percent, while the NSAID indomethacin reduced it by 54 percent.[6] A recent UCLA study confirms that ibuprofen cuts the number of plaques in the mouse model of Alzheimer's in half, delaying the effects of this disease.[7]

Numerous human studies have found that long-term use of NSAIDs is associated with a lower risk for development of Alzheimer's disease.[8] One study in particular reported this finding, in which female twins taking anti-inflammatory drugs dramatically decreased the incidence of Alzheimer's disease by approximately 75 percent.[9] Although the NSAIDs didn't work as well in men, it's still good news since women have two to three times the risk of getting Alzheimer's disease than men.

Two small studies in human postmortem tissue reported that even though patients who took NSAIDs had a shorter duration of illness, they did not have fewer plaques. In one of these studies, the amount of amyloid beta was actually increased even though deactivation and reduced numbers of damaged cells was reported, along with improvement of the patients.[10] According to the authors, this finding tends to confirm what some researchers have been saying for a long time: Reducing the number of plaques and tangles may not be as important as stopping the activation of cells creating tissue damage. So, in essence, it is important to stop the inflammatory process, not necessarily to figure out how to undo the damage that has already been done. In this study, patients were taking the NSAIDs ibuprofen (600 mg/day), ketoprophen (100 mg/day), or naproxen (500 mg/day).

Participants in the Baltimore Longitudinal Study of Aging who had a history of long-term (greater than two years) use of NSAIDs were found to have a lower relative risk for development of Alzheimer's disease, compared with those who did not have such history.[11] This study examined over 2,300 participants for fifteen years (1980–1995). Other studies that have looked at the effects of NSAIDs on Alzheimer's have reported a link between these drugs and reduction in the risk of the disease. This study, however, was the first to look at a large number of patients over a substantial period of time, as opposed to previous studies done at fixed points in time. Individuals with less than two years of NSAID use also reported a benefit. Long-term use of the common over-the-counter drugs acetaminophen and aspirin had no effect on the development of Alzheimer's disease. Preliminary results report that long-term NSAID use may slow the rate of cognitive decline in patients with Alzheimer's disease.[12]

The National Institute on Aging (NIA) is launching a clinical trial in 320 patients to determine whether treatment with certain NSAIDs will slow cognitive and clinical decline in patients with Alzheimer's disease. The study has been named the Alzheimer's Disease Anti-Inflammatory Prevention Trial (ADAPT) and is planned to begin in 2001 after patient selection. Study participants will be seventy years or older, and have a mother, father, sister, or brother who has (or had) serious age-related memory loss, dementia, senility, or Alzheimer's. Participants cannot themselves have been diagnosed with dementia, senility, or Alzheimer's. The patients will be randomized to receive either a placebo, a conventional NSAID, or a selective Cox-2 inhibitor for five to seven years. Study results, it is hoped, will be very exciting news—many treasured family members suffer from this dreaded disease.

ASPIRIN AND ALZHEIMER'S

Aspirin is technically an NSAID, but may have anti-inflammatory properties in higher dosages. It too may reduce the risk of Alzheimer's disease, although the data are not as compelling as for other NSAIDs. In an analysis of data from the Baltimore Longitudinal Study of Aging, the relative risk of getting Alzheimer's disease was reduced 26 percent by aspirin. By comparison, taking a nonaspirin NSAID two years or longer reduced it by 60 percent. However, aspirin use might have an advantage in that it reportedly produces effects similar to those of other NSAIDs in a shorter period of time. So aspirin's protective effect might kick in faster than other NSAIDs'. Better yet, a combination might work the best. Data from the Cache County Study show that combining another NSAID and aspirin works better than an

NSAID or aspirin alone. As with ibuprofen, a low dose of aspirin (81 mg) appears to be all that's needed to produce positive benefits. Most of the people in the study were taking a low dose of aspirin for cardiovascular protection.

COX-2 INHIBITORS AND CANCER

Most of us are aware that there are limitations in the current Western clinical approaches to cancer treatment. The ongoing battle against cancer has been waged for several decades—and unfortunately without much curative success from the use of chemotherapy or radiotherapy in most common solid tumors.[13] Much of the present-day research directed against active malignancies has shifted toward identification of strategies affecting the growth rate or apoptosis (cell death) of such cancerous cells so that life with cancer can be greatly extended without the harmful effects of the more aggressive therapies.

As many of the malignancies are attributable to dietary and lifestyle factors, it seems logical that changing these factors may decrease the incidence and destructive abilities of malignancies.[14] In addition, there are many environmental and chemical factors suspected of playing a role in the occurrence of malignancies, such as pollution, pesticide and preservative ingestion, cigarette smoke, and the ingestion of heterocyclic amines (found in cooked foods such as grilled meats).[15,16] With the poor success rate for treatment of most common tumors, cancer prevention is a major priority.

Colorectal cancer is second only to lung cancer as the most common cause of cancer death in the United States.[17] Both environmental (e.g., diet, physical activity) and genetic (e.g., family history, mutations, polymorphisms) factors are related to colon cancer risk. Studies have reported that regular users of aspirin and other nonsteroidal anti-inflammatory drugs (NSAIDs) may produce a reduction in risk of various cancers, including colorectal, lung, head/neck, bladder, and prostate.[18,19,20,21] A possible mechanism of this benefit is decreased prostaglandin production, which is achieved through inhibition of cyclooxygenase (Cox) activity.

Both Cox-1 and Cox-2 have been identified in conjunction with some cancers. Cox-2 is expressed in colorectal adenomas and carcinomas, both in humans and in rodents.[22] Therefore, inhibition of Cox-2 has been shown to decrease the incidence of carcinogen-induced neoplasia in rats and to lower the incidence of adenomas in the laboratory models. The identification and characterization of an inducible Cox-2 in inflammatory cells in cancer has led to the hypothesis that a selective inhibition of Cox-2 could result in relief of inflammation and pain without causing the Cox-1-dependent side effects (gastrointestinal ulceration, platelet dysfunction, kidney damage) of conventional NSAIDs. There are quite a few laboratory studies reporting the benefits and protective ability of the Cox-2 inhibitors in decreasing the risk of developing colorectal cancer and also in the treatment of these cancers.[23,24,25]

A recent study at the M. D. Anderson Cancer Center in Houston reported that one of the patented Cox-2 inhibitors was effective in reducing the number and size of colorectal polyps in patients with an inherited condition known as familial adenomatous polyposis, or FAP.[26] Patients with FAP can have hundreds or even thousands of colon polyps and are at high risk for developing colorectal cancer. This randomized, double-blind and placebo-controlled study included seventy-seven patients with FAP. Patients were randomized into treatment groups receiving 100 mg of celecoxib (Celebrex), a selective Cox-2 inhibitor, twice a day; 400 mg of celecoxib twice a day; or a placebo. Those taking 400 mg of celecoxib for six months experienced a reduction in the number, size, and overall colorectal polyp burden, defined as the sum of the polyp diameters. Moreover, there were fewer patients in this treatment group who experienced an increase in the number of colorectal polyps compared with those in the placebo group. Cox-2 inhibitors can induce early disruption of the adenoma-carcinoma sequence and may suppress subsequent cancer formation at the adenoma stage.[27]

A recent study also found that the Cox-2 enzyme might also play a role in other cancers by promoting development of blood vessels to feed tumors, further verifying the potential need for Cox-2 inhibitors in cancer therapy.[28] In recent years, cancer researchers have turned to the field of angiogenesis (development of new blood vessels) as a hopeful avenue in fighting cancer by more indirect means than traditional chemotherapy or radiation therapy. Tumors produce growth factors to recruit new blood vessels to bring the oxygen and nutrients the tumors need to grow. These vessels also provide a route for metastasis (spread of cancer cells to other parts of the body). The researchers report that lung tumors in animal models grew at a slower pace when the gene for the Cox-2 enzyme (cyclooxygenase-2) was deliberately eliminated. In addition, tumor growth was significantly reduced by treatment with a Cox-2 inhibitor in the animals that had the active Cox-2 gene. Upon closer examination, they found that in the absence of Cox-2, the tumors developed about 30 percent fewer blood vessels than those in animals whose Cox-2 gene was present and active. They also found that increasing Cox-2 levels was directly associated with increasing levels of a growth factor that promotes the development of new blood vessels. The link that is beginning to be established between Cox-2 and angiogenesis is important because it suggests that selective Cox-2 inhibitors might be useful as potential treatments for already established tumors. However, as discussed earlier, the question of whether or not Cox-2 inhibitors may increase the nutrition to tumors has yet to be answered.

DRUGS AND HOW THEY ARE MADE

Most of us are content to know that effective herbal supplements and pharmaceutical drugs are available for us when we need them. Yet we do not know very much about the remedies we take—whether synthetic or "natural." Our medicine cabinets are filled with pills for pain, indigestion, constipation, insomnia, anxiety, depression, and many other health conditions. Our society truly has a "pill-for-every-ill" mentality. But we know little about what we are taking.

An understanding of how medicines are created and what is involved in determining how safe and effective they are can help consumers have a greater appreciation for the products that are on the market and also be more responsible in the use of the potent synthetic and natural remedies that are available today.

In the past, small quantities of natural substances were used to create remedies for many different physical problems that people faced. A major problem with these early remedies was that they could not be made in a standard fashion. The same pharmacist may have made the same remedy in different ways on different occasions. And, of course, different pharmacists created different versions of the same drug. So the patient could never be sure that one batch of medicine was equivalent to the other in safety and effectiveness. In the last fifty years, increasingly sophisticated technology has revolutionized the production of medicines, but they still remain a mystery to those who take them.

The public learns most of what it knows about drugs from television, newspapers, and magazines. However, the mass media usually focus on medications that they are trumpeting as the new cure for a major disease or the new danger to public health. Public interest in health and medicine is higher than ever, but it is difficult to get reliable information.

Drugs are developed through research—that is, the search for and interpretation of new knowledge. Although there are common steps involved in the research process, each individual remedy has factors specific to it alone and so has its own unique course of development. There is no one-size-fits-all model for research when it comes to medications. However, there are components of the development process that will be part of most research. Among them are:

- Discovery
- Scientific characterization of the remedy (e.g., chemical or biological)
- Safety testing (animal studies)
- Formulation of the product
- Human pharmacological evaluation
- Human safety testing
- Human efficacy testing
- Governmental regulatory processes

In addition to the above components, once the research process has produced a medicine that seems to be valuable, each manufacturer will have its own way of going about marketing, manufacturing, supplying, and distributing the medicine to the public.

The manufacturer must be able to make an adequate amount of the product, with a sufficient degree of purity, in a formulation that delivers an effective dose of the medicine to the targeted part of the body at the correct time. This process is quite complicated and it is no small achievement when a successful medicine is created.

Every effort is made to eliminate contaminants and to reduce the number and severity of unwanted effects of the medication. However, not all adverse effects can be completely eliminated. There is always a trade-off between good and bad effects. This balance between positive and negative effects of a product is called the therapeutic ratio.

It is quite expensive to create an effective medicine and it can take a long time. And, despite years or even a decade of effort, success is not guaranteed. Substances fail at every stage of the development process. Some research indicates that only 1 in 10,000 compounds studied is successfully developed into a useful medicine. It is difficult to be precise about this figure, but it is safe to say that relatively few compounds that have been studied wind up in your medicine cabinet. Why do investors and manufacturers engage in such a risky enterprise? Because the potential earnings from a successful product can run into the billions of dollars.

DRUG DISCOVERY

Since antiquity, through trial and error, people have identified plants and other substances that have beneficial health effects, whether eaten in the natural state or cooked in some way. Alcohol is a good example of this because it was independently discovered by virtually every culture on earth. People quickly learned how alcohol affected them when taken in small, moderate, or copious amounts! Alcohol produces a continuum of effects in human beings, varying with the dosage taken and the time period involved. This general pattern applies to other drugs as well. Similarly, trial and error revealed the useful and harmful properties of many substances, such as cocaine from coca leaves and opium and morphine from poppy juice. Drug development remained in this relatively primitive state for millennia, until the modern era.

At the beginning of the modern era of drug development, research led to great progress, such as the use of vitamin C, or ascorbic acid, to prevent scurvy; the cinchona bark and quinine for malaria; willow bark and aspirin for pain and inflammation; digitalis from foxglove for cardiac problems. However, at first, drug development grew slowly. With the advent of synthetic chemical drug research, the picture changed dramatically.

In 1928, Alexander Fleming made a chance observation that led to the discovery of penicillin. This discovery did not find its full potential until World War II. In the mid-1950s, drug development exploded. Many different kinds of antibiotics were created; new anti-inflammatory drugs came to market; medications for hypertension and cardiovascular disease appeared; and tranquilizing, anxiety-reducing, and hypnotic drugs for mood disorders such as anxiety and depression were developed. The birth control pill radically changed sexual behavior. The rapid development of drugs continues to this day and, as a result, there are now more than 350,000 drugs available to consumers.

One key to the great success of the pharmaceutical industry over the past fifty years has been the vast funds it can spend on marketing and advertising. The industry spends more on promotion than it does on research. Another key to the profitability of the industry is founded in great part on the methods used to manufacture its products.

The finished products of the drug industry, in whatever form they may be, are constant between narrow limits in terms of composition, contain the active ingredients claimed on the label, are of the degree of purity stated on the label, and produce predictable results. The pharmaceutical industry produces drugs whose final physical characterization is known. This characterization consists of:

- Structural formula
- Molecular formula
- Molecular weight
- Solubility in a variety of substances
- Ultraviolet and infrared absorption spectrums
- Thin-layer chromatography
- Weight loss on drying
- Ash residue
- pH of suspension or solution
- Solvent content
- Assay

Many other specific factors are known about synthetic drugs as well; terms such as *polymorphism*, *solubility*, and *isomerism* have been defined. Skilled drug technicians use sophisticated techniques to ensure the creation of standardized, quality products. The pharmacology of these drugs in normal animals and in a variety of disease models is known. The primary and secondary effects of the drugs are determined through a wide range of investigational studies. Bioavailability, half-life, and drug distribution studies all provide further vital information. The metabolism of the products, their route of excretion from the body, and their interactions with food, other drugs, and other remedies are known as well.

The formulation of the products—the careful combination of the active drug ingredient with other inert chemical substances—is also clearly determined so that the consumer is confident that the active ingredient in the medicine is present, will be absorbed, and will affect the body as intended.

The end result of all this effort is products that consumers trust and buy in quantities and that have earned the pharmaceutical industry record profits for the past twenty years.

Part 2

What You Can Do

6

Natural Cox-2 Inhibitors and Other Natural Remedies

A number of natural remedies, including herbal Cox-2 inhibitors, offer an alternative to synthetic Cox-2 drugs. Many ancient medical traditions have long recognized the effectiveness of these remedies. In fact, herbal remedies are even found in the religious texts of antiquity, such as the Bible. In the United States, it is estimated that Americans are spending nearly $50 billion out of pocket for complementary health care. The money spent to purchase herbal remedies accounts for approximately $3 billion of that astounding figure.

HERBS: BACKGROUND AND COX-2 INHIBITION

Herbal supplements, or phytomedicines, are products containing plants, parts of plants, or plant materials that may be used for teas or extracted with solvents to make liquid extracts, capsules, tablets, or other forms of delivery to the body. Most herbal supplements recommended by pharmacists and physicians will be standardized herbal supplements. These standardized herbal products are guaranteed to contain a certain amount of one or more chemical constituents contained in the crude plant—a guarantee that you're purchasing what the label states.

Herbs are big business: U.S. annual sales of herbal supplements rose to almost $6 billion in 2000 (Information Resources Inc., Chicago). Recent reports indicate that in the United States, an estimated 70 million adults use herbal supplements regularly.[1] Likewise, over 18 percent of adults in the United States use prescription drugs concurrently with herbal or vitamin products. Some of the top-selling herbal supplements include ginkgo (*Ginkgo biloba*, used for increasing peripheral blood flow and in senile dementia, continues to have the largest market share); Asian ginseng (*Panax ginseng*, used as an "adaptogen" to help regulate the body's reaction to various stresses); garlic (*Allium sativum*, used for cardiovascular health, including high cholesterol); echinacea (*Echinacea purpurea/E. angustifolia*, used to support the immune system, especially in the prevention and treatment of colds and influenza); St. John's wort (*Hypericum perforatum*, used in the management of mild to moderate depression); and saw palmetto (*Serenoa repens*, used effectively in the management of benign prostatic hypertrophy).

Although the best-selling herbs for the past few years have seen a downward trend in sales, the largest gains in dollar sales were in soy (phytoestrogen; +116 percent), valerian (sleep aid; +71 percent), elderberry (antiviral, colds/flu; +58 percent), guarana (caffeine-containing, weight loss; +49 percent), and green tea (antioxidant, anticancer, many uses; +39 percent). However the statistics are interpreted, herbal products are in the mainstream public and are here to stay as medicinal products.

Today over 25 percent of all prescription drugs are still derived from trees, herbs, and shrubs. Isolating the bioactive constituents from plants was a natural progression in our society—the powerful healing of the earth was patentable and money could be made! The following table gives some examples of common drugs that have been isolated from medicinal plants.

European Use of Herbs

The European Scientific Cooperative for Phytotherapy (ESCOP) was formed in 1990 with the objective of producing fifty European monographs on herbs. Approximately 35 percent of all medical treatment in France and Germany uses herbal and homeopathic preparations as the primary medications. Herbal products are some of the most prescribed drugs in the European pharmacopoeias. For example, *Ginkgo biloba* accounts for 2.25 percent of all prescribed German medicines, and St. John's wort outsells Prozac in Germany for the treatment of mild to moderate depression. The Institute of Medical Statistics (IMS) estimated that 80 percent of German herbal drugs had been dispensed in pharmacies; of these, 42 percent were covered by prescription. With total sales of herbal over-the-counter drugs in the member states of the European Community estimated to be almost $6.5 billion, these products must be performing satisfactorily!

In contrast to the United States, the medical establishment in European countries such as Germany, England, and France have accepted phytomedicine

Common Drugs Isolated from Medicinal Plants

Isolated Drug	Plant	Uses
Aspirin	White willow bark (*Salix alba*)	Analgesic; antipyretic (fever lowering)
Caffeine	Coffee Shrub (*Caffea arabica*)	Stimulant
Colchicine	Autumn crocus (*Crocus sativus*)	Gout medication
Cromolyn sodium	Khella (*Amni visnagu*)	Antiasthmatic
Digoxin	Foxglove (*Digitalis lantana; D. purpurea*)	Cardiac medication
Morphine	Poppy (*Papaver somniferum*)	Narcotic analgesic
Quinine	Cinchona bark (*Cinchona* sp.)	Antimalarial
Taxol	Pacific yew (*Taxus* sp.)	Anticancer
Theophylline	Tea shrub (*Camellia sinensis*)	Bronchodilator; asthma
Vincristine	Periwinkle (*Vinca* sp.)	Anticancer

(herbal medicine) for decades. The German government approves herbal medicines based on the results of clinical and pharmacological studies. In Germany, an herbal product can be marketed with drug claims if it has been proved to be safe and effective, with the legal requirements for phytomedicines (including Good Manufacturing Practices) paralleling their pharmaceutical cousins. However, Germany requires far less paperwork and data on the proof of safety and efficacy of products than does the FDA in the United States. A special commission (Commission E) was created by the Federal Health Agency (termed Bundesgesundheitsamt) in Germany to develop over 200 monographs of commonly used plant medicines. The list of herbs now totals more than 400 monographs. The American Botanical Council of the United States has published the compilation in English. Included in the work on each plant are uses, constituents, indications, contraindications, side effects, dosage, mode of administration, duration of use, and specific manufacturing requirements. If an herbal manufacturer meets all the quality requirements in a specific monograph, or has additional evidence of a product's safety and effectiveness (which can be derived from literature, anecdotal evidence from practicing physicians, or clinical studies), then the herbal product is viewed as safe and efficacious and can enjoy the legal status of prescription and/or over-the-counter medicine.

England has a long history of supporting the use of traditional herbal remedies, with King Henry VIII signing the Herbalist's Charter in the 1540s, which granted by royal decree the right of herbalists to practice their art. Homeopathy is very widely accepted in England, with this form of medicine being the queen of England's primary care. The British Herbal Medicine Association published the *British Herbal Pharmacopoeia* in 1983. This book sets manufacturing standards for 169 herbs used in the United Kingdom. Herbal monographs are published in a companion book, the *British Herbal Compendium*, Volume 1, providing important therapeutic information, such as pharmacology, dosage, side effects, and contraindications of popular herbs.

Herbal Use in the United States

Modern allopathic (or standard) medical professionals in the United States, including physicians, pharmacists, and nurses, in the past have generally considered herbal medicine merely a reflection of folklore, myth, and outdated medical treatments. However, this opinion is changing. Ironically, the World Health Organization (WHO) estimates that over 80 percent of the world's population routinely uses and is prescribed medicines of botanical origin.

The rise in the costs of medical care in the United States has initiated changes in the attitudes of the people toward standard, or allopathic, medicine. Medical costs have risen more than fifteen fold in the past thirty years and yet only a little over 40 percent of the people are served with adequate medical coverage. The current medical costs are rising faster than inflation, and insurance costs have been unaffordable to many individuals and businesses. More than twenty-five years ago, forecasters predicted that neither decreasing nor increasing amounts of money spent on health would have any further effect on how long one could expect to live. Although modern health care has great merits and accomplishments—from transplanting organs and brain surgery to cardiac drugs—treatment with less potent medicines such as herbs may be warranted as a first line of defense. People are thirsting to become empowered to help heal themselves. But we must be educated and versed in herbs and natural therapies—their uses and safety—but also know when to turn to a health care professional.

The intent of the first U.S. Congress was to "grandfather" certain herbs ("drugs") marketed prior to 1962 from the stringent requirements of the FDA. Because most of the herbs currently used for medicinal purposes in the United States were included in the early official *United States Pharmacopoeia (USP)* and the *National Formulary (NF)*, logic should allow the use of these botanical substances as medicinal agents when prepared according to pharmacopoeial standards. However, the FDA continues to argue that herbal preparations should be considered food or dietary supplements, and that they should not be allowed to carry any therapeutic claim. The FDA has prepared a compilation of herbs and spices that are "generally regarded as safe," known as the GRAS list.

In a major advance for herbal medicine in the United States, Congress mandated under the 1992 National Institutes of Health (NIH) Appropriations Bill that the NIH organize the Office of Alternative Medicine (OAM). The OAM was developed to facilitate and conduct research on alternative or complementary forms of medicine, including herbs, for their effectiveness. Now known as the NCCAM (National Center for Complementary and Alternative Medicine), funding for the office by the federal government went from $2 million annually in 1992 and 1993 to over $50 million annually in 2000! Recently, multicenter clinical trials have begun for the evaluation of several herbs, including St. John's wort for the treatment of depression, ginkgo for its use in Alzheimer's disease, and saw palmetto for treatment of benign prostatic hypertrophy. U.S. professionals are still heavily relying on European clinical data on herbs, but development of the NCCAM will certainly improve the herbal medicine research climate in the United States in the years to come.

Herb use in the United States went through radical changes in the late 1990s. Not only did health food stores pop up in strip malls in suburbs and small towns across the country, but also many neighborhood pharmacists finally became interested in and educated in the field of herbal medicine. In November 1994, after an arduous legal battle that was aided by the support of Senator Orin Hatch of Utah and citizens across the country, Congress passed a new law called the Dietary Supplement Health & Education Act (DSHEA). For the first time in its history, Congress defined dietary supplements as vitamins, minerals, amino acids, other dietary constituents, and herbs (and standardized, concentrated, extracted, and other dosage forms of the above). More important, dietary supplements were to be considered foods, not drugs, and the people of the United States could have access to herbs for personal use.

Numerous groups are preparing herbal monographs that will eventually be incorporated into National Standards. The USP and the American Herbalists Guild both are working on Pharmacopoeia works that will contain in-depth herbal monographs on the top botanicals used in commerce in the United States. Chiropractic and naturopathic medicine, aromatherapy, homeopathy, acupuncture, and herbalism are being more widely accepted as valid medical treatments, with medical insurance beginning to cover some of these options.

Cox-2 Inhibiting Herbs

Baikal Skullcap *(Scutellaria baicalensis)*. Also known as Chinese skullcap, this herb has been used in China for over 3,000 years. In addition to its widespread use to treat facial inflammation, the herb has been employed to treat restlessness, sore throat, coughs, headaches, and chest pains. It has also been effective in treating fever, chills, nausea, vomiting, diarrhea, and indigestion.

Scientists at Barcelona University, in Spain, have demonstrated the Cox-2 inhibitory properties of this highly regarded herb. In addition, researchers in Korea, Canada, and the United States have shown that the Cox-2-inhibitory effects of skullcap make it a valuable herb for the treatment of inflammatory disorders.[2]

Feverfew *(Tanacetum parthenium)*. This plant is native to the Balkan Peninsula and has been in use in Greece since the first century C.E. In the

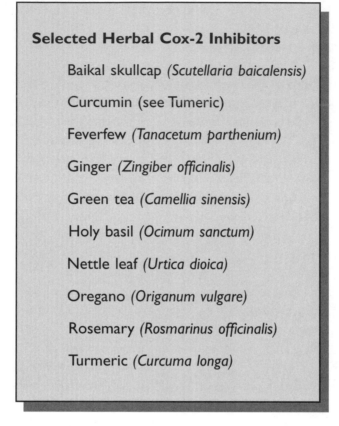

Selected Herbal Cox-2 Inhibitors

Baikal skullcap *(Scutellaria baicalensis)*

Curcumin (see Tumeric)

Feverfew *(Tanacetum parthenium)*

Ginger *(Zingiber officinalis)*

Green tea *(Camellia sinensis)*

Holy basil *(Ocimum sanctum)*

Nettle leaf *(Urtica dioica)*

Oregano *(Origanum vulgare)*

Rosemary *(Rosmarinus officinalis)*

Turmeric *(Curcuma longa)*

United Kingdom, it is widely used to treat the joint inflammation that is a painful symptom of arthritis and rheumatism. It is also widely used around the world for migraine headache, and may also traditionally be used for stomach problems, fever, and menstrual difficulties.[3]

Scientists at Louisiana State University Biomedical Research Center were among the first investigators of Cox-2 inhibitors, and they discovered that the anti-inflammatory effects of feverfew—long known to practitioners of herbal medicine—were due to Cox-2 inhibition. Since then, a growing body of research has confirmed their findings.

The recommended dosage of feverfew is 100 to 250 mg (standardized extract) one to three times a day. Products should be standardized to contain at least 0.2 percent parthenolide per dose. Warnings include:

• Use with caution in individuals with severe ragweed allergy or allergy to members of the daisy and chrysanthemum family (Compositae).

- Based on animal studies, do not use if pregnant.[4]
- Individuals on anticoagulant and antiplatelet medications and those with bleeding disorders should use with caution.[5]

Ginger *(Zingiber officinalis)*. Ginger has a legion of uses. It is primarily known in the West as a spice and as a flavoring. However, in China it has been used for thousands of years for medicinal purposes to treat such conditions as nausea, stomachache, rheumatism, and toothache. It has also long been used in Brazil, China, India, Indonesia, New Guinea, Sudan, and Thailand to treat the pain and fever associated with inflammatory disorders. Recently researchers have discovered that ginger has powerful antioxidant and anti-inflammatory effects.[6] The pharmacologically active components of gingerroot are believed to be aromatic ketones known as gingerols.

Ginger inhibits Cox-2. In experimental studies, it has been shown to inhibit both the cyclooxygenase and lipoxygenase pathways and the production of prostaglandins, thromboxane, and leukotrienes, just as the NSAIDs do. Yet its clear advantage is that no significant side effects have been reported, unlike the NSAIDs, which can have quite serious side effects associated with their use.

Ginger has 477 known constituents; synthetic Cox-2 inhibitors have one active ingredient. The secret to the success of ginger lies in the activities of its multiple and varied constituents. Ginger safely modulates Cox-2 and also balances Cox-1 enzyme processes. The evidence of ginger's anti-inflammatory effects is quite strong. In fact, many experts believe that the ancient Ayurvedic assertion that ginger is a universal medicine can be substantiated by modern science.

The recommended dosage of ginger is 250 mg (standardized extract) three times a day as needed. Products should be standardized to contain at least 5 to 20 percent gingerols per dose, most prominently being 6-gingerol and 6-shogaol, or 4 percent volatile oils per dose. Individuals on anticoagulant and antiplatelet medications, and those with bleeding disorders, should use with caution.[7]

Green tea *(Camellia sinensis)*. It is believed that green tea was discovered nearly 4,700 years ago by a Chinese emperor. As the story goes, he was in the forest, sitting down, drinking a cup of hot water, when the wind blew a leaf from the plant *Camellia sinensis* into his cup. He let it steep awhile and soon became enamored of its aroma. He drank the tea and was delighted. In addition to its use in spiritual and meditation practices, green tea is employed to help with a great variety of health problems, such as muscle aches and pains, headaches, cramps, fatigue—all of which are associated with inflammatory disorders. Recent studies report that it may protect against cardiovascular disease, has anticancer properties, and has strong antioxidant activity. In India, green tea is also used as a stimulant, a diuretic, and an astringent.

Green tea has several highly active Cox-2 inhibitors—natural salicylic acid and polyphenols.[8] Scientists in the United States, Sweden, Taiwan, Germany, and other nations have documented its effectiveness. Tea has even been reported to play a role in improving or maintaining bone mineral density.[9] Some researchers recommend that green tea be used in combination with turmeric and ginger. The recommended dosage is 250 to 500 mg (standardized extract) daily. Products should be standardized to contain between 50 and 97 percent polyphenols (the more the better), containing at least 50 percent epigallocatechin-3-gallate (EGCG) per dose. Caffeine-free products are recommended.

Holy basil *(Ocimum sanctum)*. In India this plant is called *tulsi* or *tulasi*, which in English means "matchless." References to holy basil are extremely common in Hindu literature. It was considered holy by Lord Vishnu himself, and some people actually devote their lives to its cultivation and protection. In India it was most commonly used for fever, the flu, bronchitis, asthma, malaria, and cancer. In Egypt, this herb is used for arthritis and inflammation.

Holy basil contains phytochemicals (particularly rosmarinic acid) that have reported Cox-2-inhibitory effects.[10] One study conducted at Dartmouth Medical School found that it possessed great anti-inflammatory activity. French researchers have also shown that holy basil has potent Cox-2 inhibitory effects. Studies in India and other nations around the world have confirmed these findings. Experts highly recommend this herb for the general public for a wide range of uses. An extract of holy basil has been reported to have anti-stress actions in laboratory animals, by balancing the levels of corticosteroids in the blood. It appears to help with the side effects of stress. The recommended dosage of holy basil is 400 mg daily, standardized to contain 1 percent ursolic acid per dose.

Nettle leaf *(Urtica dioica)*. In Germany, nettle leaf has a long tradition of use for arthritis. Nettle leaf extract contains a variety of active compounds (e.g., cyclooxygenase and lipoxygenase inhibitors) that affect cytokine secretion. Nettle leaf reduces the tumor necrosis factor (TNF-a) levels by inhibiting the genetic transcription factors that are involved as the condition flares up and subsides. Nettle has been used in the past for childhood eczema and gouty arthritis because of its reported ability to promote the excretion of uric acid.[11] One study of healthy volunteers reported the anti-inflammatory potential of nettle. Another study conducted on forty patients suffering from acute arthritis compared the effects of 200 mg of an NSAID with 50 mg of the NSAID combined with 50 g of stewed nettle leaf per day. Total joint scores improved by 70 percent in both groups. The results showed that nettle leaf extract clearly improved the anti-inflammatory effect of the NSAID. The addition of nettle extract resulted in a 75 percent dose reduction of the NSAID. Although much less of the drug was used, the same anti-inflammatory effect was achieved. There also were reduced side effects. Dosages are *freeze-dried leaf:* 300 to 1,200 mg; *leaf liquid extract:* 30 to 120 drops of liquid extract two or three times a day in a beverage of 1 part herb to 1 part solvent, weight to volume—1:1w/v—(fresh plant) or a 1:4w/v (dry plant) extract.

Oregano *(Origanum vulgare).* This plant is native to the Mediterranean and was used extensively by the ancient Greeks. In Greek its name means "joy of the mountains." The use of oregano spread throughout Europe, where it was frequently used to fight respiratory inflammations. It was also used as a sedative and a diuretic. In China, oregano is used for skin inflammation, digestive problems, and fever. In the United States, the medical literature shows that oregano has been used to treat arthritis, toothache, tinnitis (ringing in the ears), and anxiety.

The constituent rosmarinic acid (also found in oregano and other herbs such as holy basil and rosemary) has been reported in laboratory studies to have Cox-2-inhibiting properties comparable to ibuprofen, naproxen, and aspirin at 10-, 100-, and 1000-microM concentrations, respectively.[12] It also has the capacity to pass directly through the skin into the bloodstream, and this transdermal capability may offer a new way to apply this anti-inflammatory agent directly to the site of the problem. Both ancient physicians and chefs have long loved oregano. Its Cox-2-inhibiting properties should bring new devotees among those seeking relief from the symptoms of inflammatory disease. The recommended dosages are *leaf extract:* 250 to 500 mg, three times a day; *concentrated oil extract:* 5 to 10 drops, three times a day. Products are usually standardized to contain 5 percent thymol per dose. Allergies to oregano may develop or exist in sensitive individuals.[13]

Rosemary *(Rosmarinus officinalis).* The Latin meaning for rosemary is "dew of the sea." Throughout the ages this plant, which comes from the Mediterranean, has been used as a mental stimulant. However, it is also employed to help treat inflammations and irritations. When she was in her seventies, Queen Elizabeth of Hungary was fond of a lotion called Hungary water, which was very effective in helping fight the attacks of gout that plagued her. She applied the lotion regularly, and after a period of time she recovered fully.

Medical research is beginning to confirm rosemary's effectiveness as an anti-inflammatory. In 1992 researchers at the Medical School at the University of Limoges in France reported that rosemary had Cox-2-inhibiting properties. Swedish scientists reported in 1998 that a major constituent of rosemary possessed significant Cox-2-inhibiting effects, and researchers at Rutgers University in the United States also discovered that rosemary extracts had Cox-2-inhibiting properties.

Turmeric *(Curcuma longa)*. This herb is a "cousin" to the ginger plant. Well known as a spice, it is also used to treat systemic inflammations, skin lesions, blood disorders, chest pain, liver problems, and menstrual problems. Turmeric is widely used in the ancient Ayurvedic and traditional Chinese medical systems. Researchers at New York Presbyterian Hospital and the Weill Medical College at Cornell University have shown that one of the major phytochemicals in turmeric has potent Cox-2-inhibitory factors. Scientists at Vanderbilt University and at the University of Leicester in England have also reported that turmeric is a powerful Cox-2 inhibitor.

Turmeric contains a powerful anti-inflammatory chemical called curcumin. Studies have indicated that curcumin is about 50 percent as effective as cortisone, but it does not produce the damaging side effects of the synthetic drug—and it does not damage the pocketbook as greatly either. At high doses, curcumin stimulates the body's production of its own natural cortisone-type chemicals. Turmeric spice does not contain enough curcumin to supply the recommended dose, so supplementation is necessary. Curcumin is effective in treating gout, carpal tunnel syndrome, swelling, gallstones, and stroke. The recommended dosage is 100 to 300 mg (standardized extract) three times a day with meals. Products should be standardized to contain 95 percent curcuminoids per dose. Do not use if biliary obstruction is present.[14] Do not use unless under the supervision of a physician if on anticoagulant or antiplatelet medication or have bleeding disorders.

A New Herbal Supplement

Historically, the herbs listed in the previous section have been reported by scientific studies to have Cox-2-inhibiting properties. However, it has been reported that turmeric *(Curcuma longa)* may also inhibit the Cox-1 enzyme, which may cause gastrointestinal sensitivities in some individuals.[15] Caution should be used in those with gastrointestinal problems such as ulceration until further research is performed on this herb and others having Cox-2-inhibiting qualities. However, a new dietary supplement may be the answer for those with concerns of stomach and gastrointestinal upset.

A new dietary supplement product, Nexrutine, contains an extract of the phellodendron plant and has been reported to be helpful in the management and potential treatment of inflammatory diseases. Research has reported that phellodendron not only has Cox-2-inhibiting qualities, but also protects the gastrointestinal tract against ulceration. Phellodendron has been used for centuries in Chinese medicine for individuals with gastroenteritis, abdominal pain, and diarrhea. A Japanese study of laboratory animals with alcohol- and aspirin-induced gastric ulcers reported that phellodendron actually decreased gastric acid content, protecting the stomach lining and suppressing ulceration.[16] This is exciting news, as we now have a natural product that not only can be used for inflammatory conditions, but may also aid in protecting the stomach lining against gastric ulceration—the main problem with using NSAIDs and conventional Cox-2 inhibitors.

Nexrutine may be a viable alternative to the new synthetic "super aspirins" that are now on the market, whose sales total $1.5 billion a year. The plant on which the product is based has been used safely in China for 1,500 years. Most significant human studies show that Nexrutine blocks the "bad" chemical (95 percent inhibition of Cox-2) and does not interfere with the "good" chemical (no inhibition of Cox-1). This is very good news.

Nexrutine's mechanism of action has been reported to be different from that of other Cox-2 inhibitors. It does not act directly on the inflammatory enzymes but instead inhibits the gene responsible for the production of Cox-2 and other chemical mediators that cause inflammation. In animal studies, Nexrutine proved to be as effective as naproxen in reducing pain and inflammation.

At the time of this writing, there are two brands available that contain the Nexrutine ingredient: FlexAnew™ from Natrol and PharmaFlex™ from Puretek. As other brands include Nexrutine in their formulas, the products will be listed at www.nexrutine.com.

OTHER NATURAL REMEDIES

Glucosamine Sulfate and Hydrochloride[17,18,19]

Glucosamine is a naturally occurring substance in the body. Taken as a supplement, it is probably the best known of the natural therapies for osteoarthritis (OA). It is used extensively in Europe and recently it has become widely available in the United States.

The body uses supplemented glucosamine to synthesize substances vital for maintaining healthy cartilage. Glucosamine helps to improve flexibility and mobility in the joints. It also inhibits certain enzymes that destroy the cartilage (e.g., collagenase and phospholipase), slows the progression of the disease, and relieves symptoms for weeks after the treatment has ended.

There are many studies confirming the excellent effect and safety of glucosamine. One study evaluated 178 patients suffering from OA of the knee. Participants were divided into two groups. In one group, patients were treated for four weeks with glucosamine sulfate, 1,500 mg daily. The other group received ibuprofen at 1,200 mg per day. The data showed that glucosamine relieved symptoms as effectively as ibuprofen. In addition, glucosamine was better tolerated than ibuprofen.

Because glucosamine is a physiological substance normally used by the body, it is safe and the body is able to tolerate it. The beneficial effects of glucosamine usually take a number of weeks to appear (one to eight weeks). However, once they are achieved, they tend to last for a significant time even after treatment is halted. The recommended dosage is 500 mg, three to four times a day, with increased doses depending on severity of symptoms and tolerability of glucosamine. Individuals on sodium-restricted diets and those concerned about potassium intake should use glucosamine HCl instead of glucosamine sulfate.

Chondroitin Sulfate[20,21,22]

Chondroitin, a major component of cartilage, is mainly composed of glucosamine sulfate. Chondroitin sulfate stimulates the production of cartilage and it has the ability to prevent enzymes from destroying cartilage. The body absorbs much less chondroitin sulfate than it does glucosamine (10 to 15 percent vs. 90 to 98 percent).

Despite the differences in absorption rate, recent studies have demonstrated good results with long-term treatment using chondroitin sulfate. Patients experienced reduced pain and increased range of motion. A double-blind clinical study, which lasted for one year, was comprised of forty-two patients with OA. The researchers found that chondroitin sulfate was well tolerated, significantly reduced pain, and increased joint mobility. The quality of chondroitin does make a difference. Type IV or VI chondroitin is needed to maximize the benefits that it can have for joints.

In another double-blind study, 119 patients with finger-joint OA were followed for three years. Chondroitin was administered at a dosage of 400 mg three times daily. Significantly fewer patients developed progression of the disease in the group treated with chondroitin sulfate. These patients had a lower consumption of painkilling drugs. They also had an improved ability to tolerate the treatment.

It appears that glucosamine—as a single agent or in combination with chondroitin sulfate—is becoming increasingly recognized as the treatment of choice for OA in the United States. Because it helps to repair and improve joint function, as well as provide pain relief, this treatment offers important benefits that surpass many conventional treatments. The most common dosage is 600 mg, three times a day with meals; for maintenance, 300 mg, two or three times per day with meals.

Willow Bark[23]

Salicylic acid, first prepared from willow bark by an Italian chemist in 1838, is the basis for aspirin. Willow bark is rich in salicin and related substances that metabolize into salicylic acid. In addition to willow bark, many plants (e.g., meadowsweet and wintergreen) contain these compounds. They have a long tradition of use in Europe. Also, these products cause far fewer side effects than does aspirin.

While aspirin/salicin has been shown to have a lowering effect on some of the pro-inflammatory factors, it can also increase substances that are major inflammation-promoting mediators. One study compared the effect of aspirin alone on pro-inflammatory substances with a combination of low-dose aspirin and fish oil. The combination of fish oil and low-dose aspirin worked significantly better than aspirin alone. The recommended dosage of white willow bark supplements is 500 mg, up to three times a day, standardized to contain 7 to 9 percent salicin per dose. Do not use if allergic to aspirin and/or salicylates. Do not use in children due to potential for Reye's Syndrome. There may be interactions of white willow with other medications, so if you are taking prescription or over-the-counter medicines, ask your pharmacist or physician before taking white willow bark supplements.

Fish Oil[24]

Dietary fatty acids determine the composition of lipids in the cell membranes. This affect influences the production of chemical substances that produce and inhibit inflammation—the more balanced the intake of omega-6 and omega-3 fatty acids in the diet (whether it be through foods or supplements), the more inflammation is inhibited. It appears that omega-3 oils, such as fish oil (e.g., EPA and DHA) and flaxseed oil, can suppress the production of chemicals that produce inflammation. As a result, omega-3 oils can influence the course of chronic inflammatory diseases such as rheumatoid arthritis (RA).

In one double-blind study of seventy-eight patients with inflammatory bowel disease, an enteric-coated fish-oil preparation was used. The study ran for one year. After a year, 59 percent of the fish-oil group remained in remission. Only 36 percent in the placebo group were in remission. These results suggest that fish oils exert a significant anti-inflammatory effect.

In other investigations, dietary omega-3 oils have also demonstrated a suppressive effect on the production of substances that stimulate the production of chemicals that promote inflammation. When RA patients were given fish-oil supplementation, the results indicated that an increase of dietary omega-3 oils can be a useful adjunct to treatments for RA. A large number of studies suggest that dietary omega-3 oils help relieve tender joints, reduce morning stiffness in patients with RA, and sometimes eliminate the need for NSAIDs.

In about a dozen published double-blind and placebo-controlled studies with fish oil, researchers found decreased joint tenderness to be the most common positive result of treatment. Another three studies demonstrated that fish-oil supplementation significantly reduced the need for NSAIDs. Fish-oil consumption is not associated with gastrointestinal toxicity. Research indicates that 3 to 6 grams a day is an effective dose of fish oil. Higher dosages did not produce improved results.

Recent studies suggest that there is a potential for increased effectiveness of anti-inflammatory drugs when omega-3 oils are part of the diet. Including omega-3 oils in the diet seems to provide a safe, inexpensive way to reduce toxic side effects from RA medications. The recommended dosage of fish oils (EPA and DHA) is 500 to 2,000 mg daily. Fish oil is an omega-3 oil, which is a highly unsaturated fatty acid susceptible to oxidative damage in the body. Thus, people consuming omega-3 should take adequate amounts of antioxidant nutrients, especially vitamin E, vitamin C, and selenium. When omega-3 is purchased as a liquid, such as fish oils, it should be refrigerated to prevent it from becoming rancid. Care should be taken to minimize exposure of omega-3 fatty acids to heat, light, and oxygen. If an omega-3 fatty acid becomes rancid, it develops a bitter taste and should be discarded.

Diet

It is not widely accepted that food plays a significant role in the course of inflammatory or degenerative diseases. However, it is known that oxidative stress or free radical damage is important in the development of OA and most major chronic degenerative diseases. It is involved in aging as well.

Antioxidants are needed to fight free radical damage, and a diet rich in vegetables and fruits will add critical antioxidants to the body. However, diet alone may not always provide enough antioxidants. Vitamins C and E have been studied in their roles of supplementing these necessary antioxidants. Researchers have found them to be effective in treating OA. High doses of vitamin E, a powerful antioxidant, are reported to diminish pain. Natural foods without toxins may be more important for our health than we are now able to admit. We need to discover and test natural substances that can help the body heal and stay healthy. We need natural remedies that work in harmony with the body rather than substances that fight the body's natural functions.

Essential Oils

In her excellent new book, *The Fragrant Veil*, author Elisabeth Millar, a professional medical writer, beautifully describes the power of essential oils and demonstrates how they can be used by the reader to bring great solace and beauty into one's life. Although her book focuses on the use of essential oils to enhance and deepen sensuality and beauty, the activities she recommends are also healing, physically and emotionally. Other experts have also recommended the use of essential oils for healing, particularly for inflammation. Among those useful are black pepper, spike lavender, lemongrass, and rosemary. Either use these oils in an aromatherapy incense burner, mix with oils such as jojoba and apply topically, or just place a few drops on your temples or wrists and enjoy. Allow the aroma to calm the senses; pain relief may be realized.

CHOOSING A NATURAL REMEDY

One of the major obstacles facing consumers who wish to use natural remedies is finding products that are made according to good manufacturing procedures. There are several issues that surround the dietary supplement industry.

Product quality is the most important issue of all. It is absolutely essential that manufacturers check for the presence of contaminants such as heavy metals, pesticides, and microbes. However, this is not always the case.

These days there is a dizzying array of products for the consumer to choose from—but many of these products will not deliver what they promise because of product quality.

Traditionally, herbs were made into teas or tinctures, or were taken as raw material, and these traditional practices are the source for the herbal medical movement today. While the traditional uses of herbal products are valuable, most consumers today do not have a trained shaman to rely on to prepare their herbal prescriptions. As a result, product variability issues make it difficult to get consistent results. For the most part, consumers have had to rely on information gathered from studies that made it into the headlines or what they heard from friends. Unfortunately, there is great disparity between what is in the headlines and what is found on consumer shelves.

When studies relay the benefits of an herb, they are talking about a *specific standardized extract that is concentrated, has a guaranteed minimum percentage of active compounds, and is given in a specific dose.* For example, if you have taken aspirin to relieve a headache, you may know that it takes anywhere from 650 to 1,000 mg to gain the desired effect. If you only take 5 mg, you're probably not going to feel better.

The average consumer cannot help but be confused when trying to buy dietary supplements because product quality is so variable. Imagine you go to the store to pick up an herbal product that you heard about. If you're like most people, you shop around for the most inexpensive product, and this is a big mistake when buying herbal products. The first thing that any consumer should do is to find out what quality and strength of herb is needed in order to achieve the desired benefits. For example, if you research the herbal extract St. John's wort, you'll find that in most studies it is standardized to contain 0.3 percent hypericin. Now, even though the hypericin is not considered the active ingredient for St. John's wort, it is a product quality marker. In addition, you'll discover that 300 mg taken three times a day of a standardized extract of St. John's wort can be beneficial in relieving mild to moderate depression. But when you walk into the store, you are faced with several options.

You find a St. John's wort product in tincture or capsule form with little or no information about it or any quality studies that have been done on it. You take it for six weeks, feel no benefits from the product, and then proclaim,

"It didn't work for me." Let's say this product is named Super Mood Plus.

The next product you may choose is a standardized extract (0.3 percent hypericin), but does not have enough of an active ingredient to make a difference therapeutically because there is only 100 mg (instead of 300 mg) per capsule. You take one capsule three times a day—as the box reads—but again you proclaim, "It didn't work for me." Let's call this product Feeling Super Fine.

There is another St. John's wort product on the shelf that is standardized to a lower quality—0.15 percent hypericin instead of 0.3 percent—but it has the right amount of milligrams. Let's call this product Blues Be Gone. You take it, and again you receive little or no benefit, and again you proclaim, "It didn't work for me."

Your last option is a bottle of St. John's wort that contains capsules of 300 mg standardized to 0.3 percent hypericin. To your shock, the manufacturer is actually selling the type of extraction that was used in the studies you read that achieved a positive result alleviating mild to moderate depression.

The point of our imaginary trip to the store is that many people have tried herbs and may not have gotten the results they were looking for. But the problem may not be that the herbs don't work, but rather that contamination, reduced product quality, or incorrect dosage information or amount of ingredients may create variable results. This doesn't reflect badly on traditional herbalism, where the consumer does not shop in the drugstore for an herbal preparation but visits an expert who prepares the remedy for the individual.

Pioneering companies are taking the extra steps necessary and are committed to ensuring the quality and efficacy that are needed for the modern herbal movement to flourish. The manufacturer of Nexrutine and other remedies is one of the "good guys" in the field. Nexrutine's natural ingredients are designed for nutritional supplements, functional foods, and other natural alternatives to the over-the-counter-drug markets. The company has three areas of strength and expertise that are especially important:

1. Science-based new proprietary product development

2. Manufacturing and raw material sourcing

3. Consumer education support for products containing its ingredients

Tips on Product Choices

These are some points to remember when choosing supplements:

- Make sure the amount in each capsule or tablet is listed on the label.
- Make sure that the label indicates the standardization, or percentage of active ingredients or marker compounds contained in the herb (not simply the grams or milligrams of the herb present).
- Make sure the Latin name of the herb, along with the plant part used in the product, is listed on the label.
- Make sure the manufacturer's name and address are listed on the label.
- Ask your pharmacist or other health care provider for further information.

7

Current Treatment Options

Traditionally, the first line of treatment for most conditions has been conventional medical therapy. In the past, unless you were are already involved with a complementary health care practitioner or were knowledgeable about one of the many complementary medical approaches that are increasingly available to medical consumers, you would have seen an allopathic ("regular") doctor to help you manage your inflammation and pain. Today access to information is becoming easier, and both consumers and health care professionals are concerned with using the safest first line of defense for the treatment of these conditions.

TREATING OSTEOARTHRITIS (OA)

This condition can be quite unpredictable, both in terms of the course of its development and its severity. The good news is that OA need not become incapacitating or cause great discomfort. Today, the prognosis for OA is actually good. The basic goals of conventional treatment for this condition are to minimize pain and to preserve the normal functioning of the joints. There is no one approach that is successful. Conventional medicine uses a number of modalities in combination to tackle OA.

Pain medication is almost always used. Occupational and physical therapy are often employed to strengthen the joints. Patients are helped in devising effective ways to lose weight to remove added stress to the joints. And rest plays an important role in managing OA as well. In some cases, surgery may have to be considered when all other options have been eliminated.

It is generally considered best to begin treating OA without the use of drugs. Delaying the use of powerful drugs spares the body prolonged exposure and reduces the incidence of serious adverse side effects from NSAIDs. This is the ideal time to look to dietary supplements to improve flexibility, reduce inflammation, and improve overall joint health. For many patients, nondrug, nonsurgical interventions may bring about the desired goals: pain relief and maintenance of normal joint functioning. However, if the OA continues to progress, drug therapy can be initiated. If drug therapy fails to achieve the desired results, surgery can then be considered as an option.

Nondrug Methods

Hot and Cold Therapy. Some say the world will end in fire; some say the world will end in ice. Although no one knows how the world will end, we do know that both heat and cold can help end or reduce OA pain. Pain can be reduced by something as simple as a warm bath or shower. Warm compresses and heat lamps can reduce pain, lessen stiffness, and ease muscle tension. The use of warm wax (paraffin) baths can help relieve pain and stiffness in the fingers and feet. In addition, by using heat, you may actually increase your ability to exercise, which brings further benefit.

At other times, you may find that cold treatment is preferable to heat. If your pain and inflammation increase after activity, you may get more relief by applying ice packs. When using ice, make sure it is always wrapped in a towel and is not placed directly on the skin. If the area of the skin starts to feel numb, remove the ice. Neither ice nor heat should be used for more than twenty minutes.

The Value of Exercise. Both rest and exercise are needed to treat OA. Each individual must find the proper balance between the two. There are no hard-and-fast rules. Exercise is critical to maintaining muscle strength, joint motion, and fitness. However, when you feel aches and pains, take a rest. Don't start an exercise program on your own. Talk to your doctor to verify that a particular activity is appropriate for you at your stage of disease. It is also important to learn your exercises from a professional, such as a physical therapist, so you do things properly and don't injure yourself. And follow-ups at regular intervals are also very important so that the exercise specialist and doctor can monitor your progress.

The main types of exercises that will benefit you are:

1. Range-of-motion (ROM)
2. Muscle-strengthening
3. Endurance (or aerobic)

The purpose of ROM exercises, which are performed before a workout, is to reduce stiffness and pain, stay flexible, and improve joint functioning. ROM exercises involve moving the affected joints in every natural direction as far as they will go, without causing any pain. When doing ROM exercises, you may experience some mild discomfort.

The purpose of muscle-strengthening exercises is to keep the muscles in shape so that they give the joints greater support. One of the best forms of muscle strengthening for people with arthritis is isometric exercise. With isometrics, you push or pull against a stationary object. In this way, you can strengthen your muscles without putting stress on your joints and possibly injuring them. Many people find that improving their muscle tone through exercise causes a decrease in pain.

The purpose of aerobic activity is to improve your overall fitness. Swimming, bicycling, running, and walking are all examples of aerobic activity. Before beginning endurance exercises, you'll need to warm up. Gentle stretching and a brisk walk should be sufficient. Some forms of exercise may present the risk of further damaging cartilage affected by OA. That's why many experts promote swimming as the best form of aerobic exercise for people with arthritis. When walking or running, be sure to wear shoes that are comfortable and supportive, ones that will limit the shock of exercising to the joints.

Effective exercise may help you mentally as much as physically. Many people find that working out boosts their self-confidence. Swimming and other aquatic exercise offer great benefits and have advantages over many other forms of activity. They provide a good aerobic workout, strengthen muscles, and help keep joints flexible. Water workouts are particularly good for people with arthritis because they are much less stressful on the body and it is less likely that you may suffer an injury from falling. And don't forget—just being in the water itself has therapeutic value. Warm-water exercise is recommended for people with arthritis, and the warm water alone can reduce pain. It may take a number of months for you to see the benefits. You will get the optimum results if you can perform endurance, range-of-motion, and muscle-strengthening exercises four or five times a week.

There are public and private pools open to the public and available in almost every community. Find one near your home and try this form of self-help before popping a powerful pill. Call your local chapter of the Arthritis Foundation and ask about the instructional materials it has available to teach you about aquatic exercises.

As was mentioned earlier, rest is an essential part of your exercise program. And there is more to rest than merely avoiding activity. Other techniques for resting include wearing a sling when appropriate, using a cane, wearing a splint, and using special inserts in your shoes or wearing special shoes. Talk with your physical therapist before using any of the above aids to make sure you use them properly and don't inadvertently cause yourself additional problems.

Therapeutic Agents for OA

For many people with OA, the first analgesic or pain reliever to try is acetaminophen (e.g., Tylenol). Aspirin may also be effective, although some cannot tolerate the adverse side effects aspirin sometimes causes in the stomach. For the past two decades, nonsteroidal anti-inflammatory drugs (NSAIDs) have been widely used when acetaminophen does not bring relief. These drugs are now available over the counter in drugstores, supermarkets, and many other retail outlets. Among the most well-known NSAIDs are Advil and Motrin (ibuprofen), Aleve (naproxen), and Orudis KT and Actron (ketoprofen). Most drug chains sell effective generic versions of NSAIDs, which cost far less than the brand-name products. As previously discussed, the Cox-2 inhibitors have become available (Celebrex and Vioxx). These drugs are too new for inexpensive generic versions of them to be on the market. On rare occasions, physicians may resort to injecting an affected joint with another type of drug, the corticosteroids.

It is not unusual for a patient to have to try a number of different drugs before finding one that provides reliable pain relief without serious side effects. Each person has different biochemistry that reacts differently to these chemicals.

Acetaminophen. Inflammation is not a major concern for most people with OA. Therefore, acetaminophen may be the drug of choice. NSAIDs, which have potent anti-inflammatory effects, usually are not needed. Acetaminophen can generally provide adequate pain relief without causing any serious side effects. The maximum recommended dose of this drug is 4,000 mg daily. If you take more than the recommended dose, you can cause problems for yourself. In addition, those with liver disease can be at risk of further damage by taking acetaminophen. People who drink two or more alcoholic beverages a day should not take acetaminophen. Patients with end-stage kidney disease should also avoid using acetaminophen.

Overall, despite the known risks, acetaminophen has the lowest risk of adverse effects of all the analgesics.

Nonsteroidal Anti-inflammatory Drugs (NSAIDs). These products are the next line of treatment after nondrug methods and acetaminophen have failed to do the job adequately. OA pain and other symptoms may respond to treatment with NSAIDs, but results vary greatly from one individual to another. In my experience as a pharmacist, getting the right drug in the right amount is a matter of trial and error. It generally takes about two weeks to determine whether or not a particular NSAID is helping with OA. For most people, moderate dosages will do the job.

Long-term use of NSAIDs can produce serious side effects, such as stomach irritation, bleeding, and even ulcers. Just over 50 percent of those taking NSAIDs experience gastrointestinal bleeding to some degree. People with a history of adverse reactions to NSAIDs, or with prior history of stomach ulcers, are at high risk of adverse effects from NSAIDs. Elderly patients on corticosteroids are also at high risk. They should not take these drugs, or, if they do, must be monitored closely.

Anyone with liver problems should avoid NSAIDs—for example, people with hepatitis, cirrhosis, or alcohol addiction. NSAIDs can negatively affect the health of diabetics by lowering their blood sugar levels dramatically. Diabetics are also more likely to have kidney disease, another reason not to take NSAIDs. These drugs, including aspirin, can also be a danger to people with asthma because they can worsen that condition. Heart patients who are taking the anticoagulant warfarin also should not use NSAIDs. Together, the two drugs can cause excessive bleeding.

Among the other possible adverse effects of NSAIDs are high blood pressure, kidney damage, and increased deterioration of cartilage. Ironically, NSAIDs may also relieve pain so effectively that the severity of the under-lying condition is masked. This may cause some people to engage in exercise that is too strenuous for them, resulting in further harm to the body.

If you are taking NSAIDs long term, you should have your blood count, potassium levels, and kidney functions checked after thirty days and then at six-month intervals. After six months, you should have your liver function checked. Always report side effects such as red blood in the stool, dark black stool, fluid retention, and stomach problems to your doctor or health care provider.

You can minimize risk by taking those drugs associated with fewer side effects, such as aspirin, salsalate (Disalcid), and low-dose naproxen (Naprosyn). There are two NSAIDs that are known to produce severe side effects and they should be avoided unless others have failed—tolmetin sodium (Tolectin) and indomethacin (Indocin). You can also reduce risk by taking enteric-coated pills with meals. (These pills dissolve in the intestine and not in the stomach.)

EXAMPLES OF NUTRITIONAL SUPPLEMENTS FOR OA

Herbs and Plants

Herb/Plant Part Used	Dosage and Standardization	Cautions/ Contraindications/ Adverse Effects
Boswellia (Boswellia serrata) Gum resin[1,2]	200–400 mg, three times daily, standardized to contain 65 percent boswellic acids per dose; may use topical preparation.	Use with caution in individuals taking anti-inflammatory medications such as NSAIDs.
Grape Seed (Vitis vinifera) Seed/skin[3,4,5]	25–100mg, one to three times daily, standardized to be not less than 90–95 percent polyphenols/dose.	Use with caution in individuals on anticoagulant therapy due to platelet inhibition.
Turmeric (Curcuma longa) Root[6]	300 mg, three times daily with meals, standardized to contain 95 percent curcuminoids per dose.	Some individuals may experience GI distress or irritation when beginning use. Use with caution if peptic ulceration is present. Use with caution if currently taking anticoagulant medications.[7] Do not use if biliary obstruction is present.[8]
Evening Primrose (Oenothera biennis) Seed oil	2–8 grams daily (depending on severity of condition) standardized to contain 8 percent gamma-linoleic acid per dose.	Do not use in individuals currently on phenothiazine antipsychotics or diagnosed with schizophrenia; contraindicated in epilepsy.[9,10,11] Use with caution in individuals on the following: anticoagulants (may reduce platelet aggregation);[12] seizure medication or with seizures (may lower seizure threshold).[13,14]

Nutrients

Nutrient Used	Dosage Range	Toxicities/ Warnings/Interactions
Glucosamine (sulfate or hydrochloride)[15]	500 mg, three or four times daily.	No known toxicity or serious side effects in recommended dosages; occasional reports of mild stomach discomfort.
Methyl Sulfonyl Methane (MSM)[16]	2,000–6,000 mg daily.	No known toxicity or serious side effects in recommended dosages.
S-adenosylmethionine (SAMe)[17]	400–1,600 mg daily.	No known toxicity or serious side effects in recommended dosages.
Nexrutine	250 mg, two or three times daily.	No known toxicity or serious side effects in recommended dosages.

In addition, the FDA has approved the use of diclofenac sodium (Arthotec). In combination with another chemical called misoprostol (Cytotec), it will protect the lining of the stomach from damage caused by NSAIDs.

Cytoprotective agents may also be taken to minimize the risk of developing stomach ulcers due to the use of NSAIDs. These drugs reduce the acid content of the stomach. Among these products are the heavily advertised Prilosec, Carafate, Zantac, Pepcid, and Tagamet. All are available over the counter. However, only Cytotec has been approved by the FDA specifically to help prevent stomach ulcers that can result from taking NSAIDs. Be aware that these drugs are very expensive and produce their own side effects as well. In addition to this, the decrease in stomach acid caused by these drugs can potentially lead to the depletion of several nutrients in the body.

There are other options to help your body cope with the potential side effects of NSAIDS, aspirin, and acetaminophen. Milk thistle is an herb that protects the liver from toxin damage. Due to its hepatoprotective activity, people who are chronically on drug therapy that can damage the liver should consider periodically taking between 240 and 450 mg of an 80 percent silymarin extract of milk thistle (Silybum marianum).

Cox-2 Inhibitors. Celebrex was approved by the FDA at the end of 1998, and Vioxx in 1999. They are the new kids on the analgesic block. The jury is not in yet on their long-term effectiveness and side effects profile but they are big sellers.

A New Treatment: Viscosupplementation. This natural treatment involves taking a chemical found in the synovial fluid—hyaluronan—and making synthetic drugs derived from it. Two new viscosupplementation products have been approved by the FDA, Synvic and Hyalgan. Both work by supplementing or enhancing the synovial fluid in the joint, which acts as a shock absorber. In this way, pain is reduced. At present, this method is recommended for OA of the knee after all other approaches have failed. Synvec requires three injections over a three-week period and provides relief for about six months. Hyalgan requires one weekly injection for five weeks and also produces effects for about six months. The side effects noted so far seem to be caused by the injection and not the drug.

Topical Preparations. Although many commercial topical products don't live up to their advertising promises, they are generally safe and do not produce serious side effects. These products can cover up pain by creating either a warm or cool sensation on the skin when applied to an affected area. These items are called counterirritants. Other products contain compounds that produce direct pain relief by reducing the neurotransmitters involved in pain signals in the body. For example, some products contain capsaicin, a chemical that inhibits Substance P, which is involved in causing inflammation and pain. Some substances contain salicylates that are absorbed into the bloodstream through the skin. More and more research is being done regarding getting many different natural compounds across the skin. People who are sensitive to aspirin should be careful about using these products. If any of these products causes irritation, redness, or other side effects, you should stop using it immediately.

Surgery

This approach may be an option when all else fails. The most common procedures are:

- Arthroscopy
- Resection

- Osteotomy
- Arthodesis
- Resurfacing
- Arthroplasty (total joint replacement)

Orthopedic surgeons perform arthroscopy, either in an outpatient setting or in a hospital. The surgeon uses a thin, lighted tube (arthroscope) to peer right into the affected joint. This procedure can be performed on the hips, knees, shoulders, wrists, and elbows. It can be used for both diagnosis and treatment. The complication rate is only 1 percent.

With resection, which is most frequently used for rheumatoid arthritis (RA) patients, all or part of a bone is removed. This can be done in the ankles, toes, hands, wrists, and elbows. It usually takes many weeks to recover from this surgery.

An osteotomy is performed in OA patients to remove bone that is causing joints to be out of alignment. The damaged bone and tissue are cut and removed. The remaining bone is reset. This approach is used most often with physically energetic people who want to continue activities that are high impact. Full recovery takes about six months.

With arthrodesis, two bones are fused together, usually in the foot, finger, ankle, or wrist, to form one new bone. This technique is an alternative to joint replacement for patients whose physical condition rules out replacement.

Resurfacing is also known as bone relining. It is a form of joint replacement. It involves removing the bone ends and damaged cartilage and capping them with metal. Sometimes plastic is used to cap the joint capsule.

Arthroplasty, or total joint replacement, is usually done with the hips and the knees (80 to 90 percent of procedures involve these sites). About 150,000 such surgical procedures are performed in the United States annually, mostly because of arthritis. Hip replacement is the most common operation and has a 95 percent success rate for a period of five to ten years.

You should always exhaust all other possible options before considering surgery. But if you do not respond to other therapies, if pain keeps you awake at night, if you cannot walk more than one block, and if there is evidence of further deterioration, talk to your doctor about this procedure. It is a very serious decision that requires discussion with your primary care doctor, your surgeon, other knowledgeable professionals, and, of course, your family.

In the Pipeline

Current treatments for OA provide only relief of symptoms. There is nothing available at present either to prevent the disease or to repair joint damage. However, there is research under way on approaches that may actually help repair damage or halt the progress of the disease.

The media recently have devoted a good deal of attention to glucosamine and chondroitin sulfate. These substances occur naturally and are involved in cartilage formation. The results so far are promising. (Other research involves what are called disease-modifying drugs for osteoarthritis (DMOADs.) These drugs have the potential to bring relief by limiting the production of chemicals in the body that damage cartilage. In addition, some are looking into cartilage transplants, but much more information is needed about the effectiveness of this technique. There is also much work being undertaken in the area of gene therapy for OA, but it is all still highly experimental.

TREATING RHEUMATOID ARTHRITIS (RA)

Here the goals are similar to those for OA—relieving pain, reducing inflammation, preventing deformity, and maintaining normal body functioning. A mix of medicines and other regimens are available to achieve these goals: acetaminophen, aspirin, NSAIDs, Cox-2 inhibitors, ice application, and exercise. In the near future, through the use of a functional medicine approach (e.g., addressing the problem of food intolerances, reducing overactive immune responses, handling harmful environmental influences), great strides could be made in handling these problems. Interestingly, contemporary research indicates that a positive attitude can do a lot to improve the situation among those suffering from RA. If the condition is caught early, treatment can reduce the risk of developing osteoporosis, which affects nearly 50 percent of RA patients. To date, topical preparations have had little success in treating RA.

Fatigue is a serious problem for those with RA. In fact, it can often be the most debilitating aspect of the condition. It is imperative that patients find effective ways to cope with the weariness they begin to experience (e.g., using splints to help rest inflamed joints). Also, there is increasing attention being paid to the psychological factors involved with RA and to the emotional elements that cannot be overlooked if treatment is to succeed.

Rest

Inflamed joints can suffer further damage easily. Rest is vital to prevent additional harm. And rest will reduce inflammation as well. There are four generally recognized ways to give joints the proper amount and kind of rest:

- For fifteen minutes at a time several times a day, relax, lie facedown, and then stretch your hips and knees.
- Make sure you do not sit in a flexed position too long.
- Help diminish muscle pain and spasm, and reduce development of deformity, by using splints for inflamed joints.
- Use crutches to take weight and pressure off inflamed joints.

To help relieve fatigue, it is recommended that you:

- Get a minimum of ten hours of sleep daily (e.g., eight hours at night, two through naps during the day).
- Get relief for pain immediately.
- If you have a flare-up, postpone nonessential activities.
- Focus on the tasks of the day and consolidate your activities so you don't waste energy.
- Always factor in time for rest periods between your various daily activities.

Exercise

Exercising in water is excellent for helping reduce the symptoms of RA. If your joints are inflamed, perform only passive ROM activities. After any inflammation subsides, you can begin to try more strenuous exercises. If you find that your pain increases an hour after exercising, stop performing that exercise. Moderate regular exercise is necessary to help control pain and reduce inflammation.

Helpful Devices

When inflammation flares up, pain can be relieved and joints stabilized by the use of splints, either custom made or purchased over the counter. Today, lightweight splints are available that do not inhibit range of motion. These products are easy to put on and take off. Splints designed for the hands or wrists are usually more effective than those for the hips and knees. It is important to use these devices properly because misuse can result in greater pain and muscle atrophy. For the shoulder and the elbow, drug therapy and physical therapy are preferred over splints because use of the devices can result in loss of mobility in these parts of the body. In addition to splints there are many other devices available to help with common tasks such as turning the faucets on and off and opening jars. Consult an occupational therapist for expert advice on what devices are available to help you.

Therapeutic Agents for RA

NSAIDs. Aspirin is generally the first drug recommended for reducing inflammation. It is well known, effective, and costs far less than the other NSAIDs. If you have had problems with aspirin in the past, tell your doctor. If the pain is too severe for aspirin to handle, you may have to try one of the many other NSAIDs available, such as ibuprofen and naprosyn, to control symptoms. If these drugs do not help, you may want to try one of the new Cox-2 inhibitors. No one product has proved itself to be the most effective drug for most people. Each patient must find which chemical works best in his or her body through experience.

Antirheumatics. In medicine today, the general mood is to move RA patients quickly to more powerful synthetic antirheumatic drugs. These products are called either disease-modifying antirheumatic drugs (DMARDs) or slow-acting antirheumatic drugs (SAARDs).

Antimalarial drugs are frequently employed to treat RA—for example, hydroxychloroquine sulfate (Plaquenil). This drugs helps 30 to 40 percent of RA patients, but it can take as long as three to six months before the medication begins to take effect. There is a risk of damage to the retina with this drug so the eyes must be monitored regularly during long-term therapy. Patients may also experience some gastrointestinal problems.

Another drug that offers some help is azothioprine (Imuran), a product generally used to help prevent rejection after kidney or heart transplants (termed immunosuppressive). This drug is employed only after all other standard treatments have failed to bring improvement, because it can cause major problems in the immune system. In addition, this drug can take a number of months to have an effect on RA.

Prednisone and other corticosteroids are drugs that reduce inflammation dramatically. They are also powerful immune suppressants. These drugs can produce significant side effects, especially when used long term, yet physicians and patients often resort to them for relief as a matter of necessity. Because the side effects are so serious, the American College of Rheumatology has developed a set of guidelines for their use, focusing particularly on the risk of developing osteoporosis from long-term steroid use. Most experts recommend that steroids be used only short term for acute flare-ups of RA.

Another immunosuppressant drug used to prevent transplant rejection that may help with RA is cyclosporin. By inhibiting the immune system, this drug reduces the inflammation that affects joints and causes pain. Sometimes cyclosporin is combined with an anticancer drug called methotrexate, and this improves the situation for some people.

Methotrexate was first employed in the treatment of cancer. Today it is considered by many to be the drug of choice for those who are not helped by NSAIDs. Improvement can be seen in as little as one month. But methotrexate can damage the stomach, cause liver damage, result in bone marrow suppression, or, in rare instances, cause life-threatening toxic reactions. There is even some chance that the drug may be linked with increased risk of leukemia or lymphoma. While treatment showed dramatic results in the first two years (44 to 51 percent of patients improved), that figure dropped to only 29 percent when the drug was given to people who had suffered from RA for more than five years. This suggests that the use of potent drugs is more effective in the early stages of RA.

Research conducted in the United Kingdom suggests that penicillamine may be effective for patients who do not respond to other treatments. However, because just over 50 percent of those people taking the drug suffer serious side effects, its use is limited.

Another drug that may be beneficial is sulfasalazine (Azulfidine-EN-tabs), an immunosuppressant, anti-inflammatory agent. This drug takes about one month to show any positive effects. Because it produces serious adverse effects, anyone taking the drug needs to be monitored closely during the first three months of therapy.

Experimental studies of one anticancer drug have shown that it may be of help to some RA patients. Cyclophosphamide (Cytoxan) can be effective for some who have not responded to other forms of treatment. This drug can cause serious bladder inflammation, so anyone taking it must drink plenty of water to prevent this problem. Pregnant women or women who think they may be pregnant should not take this chemical because it will cause fetal damage.

If you do not respond to NSAIDs, you may be a candidate for gold salt therapy. This agent helps about 60 percent of RA patients. As with some other drugs, benefits may not be seen for three to six months. Serious side effects occur in about 33 percent of patients using this form of treatment. Inflammation of the skin, the mucous membranes, and the stomach may occur. It is important to have regular blood tests if you are on gold salt therapy.

In the Pipeline

The currently available drugs treat the symptoms only. Researchers are trying to find medications that will affect the underlying disease process. Lately much attention has been paid to TNF (tumor-necrosis factor), a chemical that normally fights infection but which, in RA patients, produces inflammation and joint pain. The FDA has approved Etanercept (Enbrel) to minimize the inflammatory response. This drug can be used in combination with many other drugs used for RA. The FDA has also approved leflunomide (Arava) for RA patients. This is the first oral treatment for joint damage, and it also fights inflammation. This drug absolutely must not be used by pregnant women or premenopausal women who are not taking oral contra-ceptives. The drug may cause liver damage, hair loss, rash, or diarrhea. There is not enough information available on the safety and effectiveness of combining leflunomide with other drugs used to treat RA.

Some of the more promising natural agents that have recently been researched are plant sterolins, which are compounds that help to modulate the immune system. This means that if the immune system is working too hard, the plant sterolins can help it to scale back activity; or if it is not working hard enough, they help support the immune system by increasing or improving the immune response. The most heavily studied of these extracts is a product called moducare. Keep in mind that moducare will not have direct impact on pain, flexibility, or other aspects of joint function. But it should be considered as one of the options in a comprehensive approach to treating RA that includes nutritional supplements.

Surgery

The same techniques used for OA patients may help RA patients. In addi-tion, synovectomy—the removal of inflamed joint lining or synovium—can help some patients. The surgery does not result in a permanent solution because the synovium grows back over time. If medication does not succeed in controlling the disease, the problem will recur even after surgery.

EXAMPLES OF NUTRITIONAL SUPPLEMENTS FOR RA

Herbs and Plants

Herb/Plant Part Used	Dosage and Standardization	Cautions/ Contraindications/ Adverse Effects
Boswellia (Boswellia serrata) Gum resin[18,19]	200–400 mg, three times daily, standardized to contain 65 percent boswellic acids per dose.	Use with caution in individuals taking anti-inflammatory medications such as NSAIDs.
Grape Seed (Vitis vinifera) Seed/skin[20,21,22]	25–100 mg, one to three times daily, standardized to be not less than 90–95 percent polyphenols/dose.	Use with caution in individuals on anticoagulant therapy due to platelet inhibition.
Evening Primrose (Oenothera biennis) Seed oil	2–8 grams daily (depending on severity of condition) standardized to contain 8 percent gamma-linoleic acid per dose.	Do not use in individuals currently on phenothiazine antipsychotics or diagnosed with schizophrenia; contraindicated in epilepsy.[23,24,25] Use with caution in individuals on the following: anticoagulants (may reduce platelet aggregation);[26] seizure medication or with seizures (may lower seizure threshold).[27,28]
Holy Basil (Ocimum sanctum)[29]	400 mg daily, standardized to contain 1 percent ursolic acid/dose.	Use with caution if taking steroidal medications.
Olive Leaf (Olea europaea)	250–500 mg, one to three times daily, standardized to contain 15–23 percent oleuropein per dose.	Do not use in individuals with gallstones due to cholagogue effect.[30] Use with caution in individuals on hypoglycemic and antihypertensive agents.

EXAMPLES OF NUTRITIONAL SUPPLEMENTS FOR RA

Nutrients

Nutrient Used	Dosage Range	Toxicities/ Warnings/Interactions
Glucosamine (sulfate or hydrochloride)[31]	500 mg, three or four times daily	No known toxicity or serious side effects in recommended dosages; occasional reports of mild stomach discomfort.
Shark Cartilage	3,000 mg, three times daily, taken twenty minutes before meals.	Nausea is the most frequent side effect.
Methyl Sulfonyl Methane (MSM)[32]	2,000–6,000 mg daily	No known toxicity or serious side effects.
S-adenosylmethionine (SAMe)[33]	400–1,600 mg daily	No known toxicity or serious side effects in recommended dosages.
Vitamin B_5 (pantothenic acid)	10–50 mg daily	Generally safe at high doses.
Vitamin E	200–400 IU daily	When taking anticoagulant or antiplatelet medications, or if you have altered bleeding times, use only under the supervision of a physician.
Nexrutine	250 mg, two or three times daily.	No known toxicity or serious side effects in recommended dosages.

TREATING GOUT

The key to treating gout is preventing an attack from occurring. A lot is known about how to prevent flare-ups of this condition. It is also very important to prevent the buildup of urate deposits in the kidneys and to prevent kidney stones.

The Role of Diet in Treatment

Purines are chemicals that convert to uric acid. Many different kinds of food contain purines, and it used to be thought that gout was caused primarily by eating foods rich in purines (e.g., sweetbreads, kidney, liver). It is now known that limiting or avoiding such foods does not have much impact on gout. Most experts recommend maintaining a healthy weight, avoiding or minimizing alcohol consumption, and drinking enough water to produce two liters of urine daily. Fasting to control weight actually backfires because it increases uric acid levels in the body.

Drug and Nutrition Therapy

Two drugs are used to lower uric acid levels in the blood: uricosuric agents and allopurinol (Zyloprim). The uricosuric drugs increase the excretion of uric acid. Allopurinol inhibits the production of uric acids by the body. In general, if you have low levels of uric acid, your doctor will recommend that you use uricosuric agents. With higher levels, allopurinol will be selected. These drugs do not help while an attack of gout is taking place, and neither type of drug should be used during an attack. By lowering uric acid levels, these drugs can help prevent gout. Another agent, colchicines, may also be used after treatment with allopurinol has begun. Allopurinol may cause rashes and possibly even a fatal skin disorder. If you take this drug, have any rash examined immediately. Liver toxicity has also been reported with the use of allopurinol.

Colchicine can reduce the frequency of gout attacks. This drug does not lower blood uric acid levels. It seems to work best with patients who have high uric acid levels and frequent attacks of gout. It is generally used along with an antihyperuricemic drug. Drug therapy to lower uric acid levels can sometimes start an attack of arthritis and colchicines can be useful in treating the arthritis. The drug can produce rare but life-threatening side effects from allergic reactions. Nausea and vomiting, diarrhea, and stomach pain are common side effects.

Acute gout attacks are best treated by bed rest and NSAIDs. Colchicine may help early on in an attack. Corticosteroids may be used if a person does not respond to NSAIDs. Your physician may decide that narcotic analgesics may be necessary while waiting for the other analgesics to take effect. The use of cherry juice concentrate has been recommended for years by natural medicine practitioners if a gout attack is suspected of coming on. Cherries are rich in flavonoids, which can block the inflammation response and inhibit the potential for a full-blown attack. Natural therapies that can be used include anti-inflammatory herbs such as turmeric, boswellia, and holy basil, along with antioxidants and vitamins. Also, stinging nettle leaf *(Urtica dioica)* has been reported useful in ridding the body of excess uric acid.[34] Dosages are: *freeze-dried leaf:* 300 to 1,200 mg; *leaf liquid extract:* 30 to 120 drops of liquid extract two or three times a day in a beverage of 1 part herb to 1 part solvent, weight to volume—1:1w/v—(fresh plant) or a 1:4w/v (dry plant) extract. Nutraceuticals to support the bones and joints may also be used, such as glucosamine, shark cartilage, and MSM.

TREATING FIBROMYALGIA

There is no one definitive cause known for fibromyalgia. In fact, depending on the individual, there could be several causes. Some research indicates that fibromyalgia is the result of a reduction in the hormone relaxin. Other literature reports that this condition is a metabolic imbalance that is due to the inability of cells to fully burn lactic acid as fuel for the body. This results in muscle soreness and fatigue. The process could involve the adrenal glands, thyroid gland, low magnesium status, and even the functional health of the intestines. Yet another popularly held theory is that a deficiency in serotonin causes fibromyalgia. The truth is that several aspects of biochemistry are involved at the same time. As usual, the problem has been trying to isolate one cause for a most complex disorder. When you free yourself from that way of thinking, a whole new highway of hope opens up. One thing is for certain: Every fibromyalgia patient wants to be able to reduce pain and improve the quality of his or her sleep. Therefore, finding an agent to help reduce stiffness and soreness should be a primary goal no matter what individualized treatment is developed.

Exercise is essential to the improvement of fibromyalgia. The symptoms become worse with inactivity. But because of the serious fatigue that accompanies fibromyalgia, it is difficult for people with this condition to begin to exercise. However, you can start with something as simple as walking briskly for five to ten minutes a day. Over time, this can be increased to thirty or forty minutes, three times a week. Swimming is an excellent form of exercise for those with fibromyalgia. Magnesium malate supplementation could help the fatigue and the muscle soreness that come with an exercise regimen. The typical dose is 1,200 to 2,400 mg per day. Magnesium malate can cause loose stools. People who have fibromyalgia and irritable bowel should note that they must slowly work up to a therapeutic dose because it may irritate the bowel.

It is also important to establish regular sleep habits. Get at least eight hours of sleep a night; avoid alcohol, smoking, and caffeine in the evening; and resist napping during the day. If this doesn't work, medication may be needed. Your doctor can refer you to a physical therapist who will help you develop a regular exercise plan and teach you how to improve your body mechanics for everyday activities to prevent added stress to the body.

In my experience, massage therapy, acupuncture, and other complementary therapies may provide additional value and should be explored. There is an emotional component to this disorder and psychological counseling can also be of great value. Many people with this condition are also suffering from depression. The physical symptoms are real. But talking about your feelings can help, as can antidepressants if necessary.

Inflammation is not part of the picture with fibromyalgia and, therefore, NSAIDs and other anti-inflammatory drugs are not routinely prescribed. At times, acetaminophen or low-dosages of NSAIDs may be helpful. Nutritional supplements should include turmeric, cat's claw, cordyceps (a unique fungus; 1,050 mg, two times a day, standardized to contain 0.14 percent adenosine and 5 percent mannitol per dose; use with caution if taking anticoagulant or antiplatelet medications), and kava kava (used for anxiety and as a skeletal muscle relaxant; 100 to 250 mg, one to three times a day as needed, standardized to contain 30 percent kavalactones per dose; do not use in individuals with Parkinson's disease; use with caution if drinking alcohol, driving, or operating heavy machinery; do not use in pregnancy; not recommended if taking prescription antianxiety or sleep agents).

TREATING BURSITIS

This condition can be treated safely and effectively by you at home. The affected area requires rest as the first line of treatment. It is also necessary to avoid the activity that brought on the attack in the first place. Pain and swelling in the area affected can be treated with ice packs, twenty minutes at a time, for one to two hours. After two days, heat should be used to treat the affected area. This will increase the flow of blood and reduce pain. Aspirin or NSAIDs can also provide relief. Acetaminophen does not reduce inflammation and is not useful. Some natural therapies that can be used include anti-inflammatory herbs such as turmeric, boswellia, and holy basil, along with antioxidants and vitamins. Nutraceuticals to support the bones and joints may also be used, such as glucosamine, shark cartilage, and MSM.

After the attack has passed, gentle stretching exercises are recommended. Gradually build your strength back to normal levels. If bursitis pain lasts for more than three or four days, call your doctor.

TREATING DYSBIOSIS

It is also important to consider the health of the intestinal tract when dealing with dry eye syndrome, a by-product of dysbiosis. Dysbiosis is defined as a condition where harmful or pathogenic gut flora inhabit the colon. The by-products of their metabolism, along with their direct effects on the intestinal lining, may impact homeostasis. These organisms are generally of low intrinsic virulence, but alter the metabolic function or immunologic responses of their host. Consider the fact that the average child in the United States has taken multiple rounds of antibiotics in the first five years of life, with little if any replacement of beneficial flora. The impact of antibiotics on gastrointestinal (GI) flora sets up a pattern of poor absorption of nutrients, which, coupled with a poor diet, exacerbates poor absorption.[35]

In addition, this dysbiotic phenomenon can lead to leaky gut syndrome, a condition implicated in IgG-, IgA-, and IgM-mediated allergic responses leading to dry eyes. Mucosal dysfunction of the intestines may lead to abnormal absorption of intraluminal antigens. Since approximately 40 percent of the immune response in a healthy individual is initiated in the intestines, allergic responses in the gut may result in reduced immunity. The simple recommendation of probiotics with antibiotic prescriptions could have a positive benefit on a patient's overall health.

Immune response and poor nutrient absorption are factors that should be considered in an evaluation process in the treatment of inflammation. Nutrient deficiencies in chromium, magnesium, calcium, and essential fatty acids may also play a role in the symptom picture. Endotoxins secreted by unfriendly organisms may also have an impact on the neuro-logic, immune, and other metabolic functions in the body. If the patient has been or will be on antibiotics, this protocol is extremely important in decreasing the incidence of gastrointestinal imbalances.

A regimen of supplements useful in managing dysbiosis include:

L-Glutamine. This amino acid aids in nourishing the normal micro flora of the gastrointestinal tract (GIT) and decreasing bowel hyperpermeability.[36] Dosage is up to 2 g daily.

Olive leaf *(Olea europaea)*. Olive leaf is an excellent antibiotic, antifungal, and antiviral agent, helping restore the normal microflora of the GIT[37]. The recommended dosage is 250 to 500 mg, one to three times a day, standardized to contain 10 to 23 percent oleuropein per dose (most prod-ucts in the United States are 10 to 12 percent oleuropein). Based on laboratory animal studies, use with caution in individuals on hypoglycemic medications along with ACE inhibitors and other antihypertensive medica-tions.[38] Based on pharmacology, use with caution in individuals on antico-agulant and antiplatelet medications and those with bleeding disorders.[39]

Acidophilus–*Lactobacillus acidophilus, L. bifidus*. This helps promote a healthy digestive tract and is useful in dysbiosis. Use 10 to 15 billion CFU/g, two times daily. Make sure acidophilus products are refrigerated and are guaranteed to contain the recommended live bacteria.

Cat's-claw *(Uncaria tomentosa)*. Cat's-claw is reported to have the ability to soothe irritated and inflamed tissues and help eliminate pathogens from the GI tract.[40] Cat's-claw reportedly positively affects the immune system and acts as a potent free radical scavenger.[41] The recommended dosage is 250 to 1,000 mg, three times a day, standardized to contain not less than 1.3 percent pentacyclic oxindole alkaloids and not more than 0.06 percent tetracyclic oxindole alkaloids, and 15 percent total phenols per dose. Based on pharmacology, use with caution in individuals on anticoagulant and antiplatelet medications and in those with bleeding disorders.[42] Based on pharmacology, use with caution in individuals on nonsteroidal anti-inflam-matory drugs due to increased chances of GI bleeding. Based on pharma-cology, do not use in individuals on hyper-immunoglobulin therapy, passive vaccines, and immunosuppressant therapy.[43]

Grapefruit seed *(Citrus paradisi)* **extract.** Grapefruit seed extract has been reported to be an excellent broad-spectrum antimicrobial agent both *in vitro* and *in vivo*.[44] The recommended dosage is 100 mg, one to three times a day with meals. *Liquid:* 5 to 10 drops, two or three times a day with meals. *Oral rinse:* 5 to 10 drops in water, two or three times a day; swish and expectorate.

Digestive enzymes. Hypochlorhydria has been correlated with family histories of allergies.[45] Typically, betaine HCl is given along with other digestive enzymes to reduce IgE response to certain provoking foods. Recommended dosage is 1 tablet with meals.

8

A Smorgasbord of Ways to Manage Your Pain

Inflammation causes pain and pain interferes with living. *However, you have the power to control your own pain. And you do not always need medication to do this.*

About 80 million Americans suffer from chronic pain and spend over $100 billion each year seeking relief from that pain. In the last decade, there has been a consistent effort on the part of a growing number of medical professionals to deal with chronic pain. Today there are over 1,000 pain clinics in the United States using physical and psychological techniques to relieve pain.

There is no one treatment, method, or technique you can use that will help you control your pain at all times. Any one of the following suggestions may help you at some time or another. And there are far more ways than those listed below to fight pain. Use your own creativity and combine some of the pain-fighting suggestions in this book or use them as starting points from which you can develop your own pain-control techniques.

WHAT IS PAIN?

Pain is defined by *Steadman's Medical Dictionary* as "suffering, either physical or mental; an impression on the sensory nerves causing distress, or when extreme, agony." Pain is carried along two pathways through special nerve fibers. One pathway involves sensations of sharp pain, the other sensations of dull pain. If you prick your hand, you will feel pain that moves along the pathway that conducts sharp pain. If you pinch yourself, you will feel pain that moves along the pathway that conducts dull pain.

Pain depends on two factors: a stimulus and state of mind. For example, if you are expecting pain, your state of mind may actually contribute to making the pain feel worse. If you are intensely involved in an activity—on the job or playing a sport—you may not even notice an injury until you stop the activity.

Some researchers have concluded that pain is not even something that happens in the injured part of your body! Pain may not be something that happens in the nerve fibers that transmit the pain signals. It seems that *pain is something that happens in your brain.* The impulses transmitted along the pain pathways in your nervous system are translated into conscious pain sensations in your brain.

The brain interprets pain signals. This process of interpretation holds the key to your perception of pain. How pain is perceived varies greatly from person to person. It is also affected by cultural, social, and economic factors. In other words, pain is an extremely subjective phenomenon.

There are three basic kinds of pain:

1. *Nociceptive* pain involves the activation of pain-sensitive fibers in your body. This type of pain is usually felt as an aching or sense of pressure.
2. *Neuropathic* pain is not well understood. It is caused by damage to the pain pathways and is felt as a burning sensation.
3. *Psychogenic* pain is real pain; it does not include faking or malingering. This pain is usually chronic and has no identifiable organic cause. It is a *psychophysiologic* disorder.

TREATING PAIN

For most people, pain is not a disease in and of itself. The primary aim of medical treatment is to remove the cause of the pain. Treatment to relieve the pain itself is secondary. And the most effective medical treatments usually combine both physiological and psychological approaches.

Many of the pain-control techniques now used in traditional Chinese medicine were known more than 5,000 years ago. Over 4,000 years ago ancient Egyptians used morphine to control pain. In India and South America, primitive tribes have long used willow leaves to fight pain. (Willow leaves contain salicylic acid—the precursor of aspirin.) The Incas used coca leaves and the Romans used a combination of opium and wine. Even some "alternative" methods date back to the ancients. Even Plato and Aristotle discussed an ancient form of the modern electrical technique for pain control (called TENS or transcutaneous electrical nerve stimulation). It involved using an electric fish to fight both gout pain and headache. The Roman emperor Nero's surgeons also used this method.

Pain control generally involves some combination of the following five factors:

1. Interrupting pain messages before they start
2. Limiting the intensity of the pain
3. Blocking pain messages
4. Limiting pain perception
5. Controlling the pain experience

Drug therapy (non-narcotic or narcotic medications); anesthesia; physiatrics, (i.e., physical therapy with or without the use of prosthetic or orthotic devices); psychological techniques, such as hypnosis, distraction, cognitive therapy, biofeedback, relaxation techniques, supportive group therapy, and support groups; therapy with medical devices (e.g., TENS); and pain clinics are all part of effective pain treatment.

Self-help techniques can also be invaluable in fighting chronic pain. Although pain involves intricate and complex metabolic and neurologic processes in your spine and nervous system, what goes on in your brain plays a critical role in the type and intensity of pain you feel. How you think about your pain can determine how much pain you feel. Your mind can either magnify or reduce your perception of pain. One of the most crucial facts that cognitive therapy has proved is that you can control what you think. As a result, you can have some control over your pain.

In his excellent book *Free Yourself from Pain*, Dr. David A. Bresler puts forth five thoughts that can help you help yourself in your effort to control your pain:

1. All pain is real.
2. Your attitude is the key to success.
3. Your mind can be your best pain reliever.
4. You can develop your own pain plan.
5. You *can* control your pain.

The suggestions for managing your pain contained in this book can help guide you along the path to reducing your chronic pain and increasing your pleasure in life.

Sex—A Potent Pain Reliever

Sex stimulates the production of endorphins as well as cortisone, adrenaline, and other hormones. Many of these substances have anti-inflammatory effects that can reduce your pain for hours or even days at a time.

Physical pain from arthritis and other inflammatory disorders will often dampen or eliminate sexual desire. You may feel depressed in the early stages of your disease or when it flares up after a period of remission. This will lower your libido. You may also experience changes in your appearance that make you feel less desirable and cause you to fear that your partner is no longer attracted to you. That's the bad news.

The good news is that when pain is controlled, the depression usually lifts. Sharing your feelings about your body image with your partner or with your physician can help you regain a positive outlook. You may find that your interest in sex returns and that lovemaking and intimacy make you feel better, boost your confidence, and reduce your pain.

Deep Breathing

Chronic inflammatory disorders like arthritis cause muscle tension. Increased muscle tension heightens pain. Many easy-to-learn psychological and stress management techniques can help break this pain cycle. One of the simplest is deep breathing.

Pick a time when no one will interrupt you. Select a quiet and comfortable place. Put the lights down low, sit in a cozy chair or lie down on a comfortable bed. Close your eyes and rest your hands on your lap or by your sides. Breathe slowly, in and out. Establish an easy rhythm to your breathing, inhaling through your nose, exhaling through your mouth. Focus all your attention on your breathing. Let other thoughts and worries just drift away. Don't fight them—just focus on your breathing.

You may want to say a simple word like *peace* or *relax* with each exhalation. Start gradually. At first, do this about five minutes at a time. (It may not be as easy for some as it sounds at first. It can be difficult to deal with all that "noise" in your mind.) Over time, work your way up to sessions of fifteen or twenty minutes. At the end of each session you will feel lighter, less tense, and more relaxed, and your pain should be diminished.

Information Is Power

About 400 years ago the philosopher Francis Bacon wrote, "Knowledge is power." The Arthritis Foundation estimates that up to 50 percent of people with arthritis don't know what type they have. Do you know what type of arthritis or other condition you have? It helps to learn about your disease. Knowledge will help you be a partner with your doctor and take control over your own health. Ask your doctor to recommend material for you to read about your condition and your treatment. Or else call the Arthritis Foundation's toll-free number: 1-800-283-7800. Ask questions and don't settle for answers you don't understand. If your doctor has trouble dropping his or her "medicalese," don't give up. Ask for an explanation in plain English. Knowledge is a powerful tool you can use in your fight against inflammatory disorders and the pain they cause.

The Medium Is Massage

Massage can often be effective in reducing pain. It is used primarily for muscle stiffness and spasm but it also lowers pain in ways not yet completely understood. Massage produces increased blood flow to the area being massaged and that part of your body begins to feel warmer. Some feel that the pleasing sensations produced by massaging compete with the painful sensations produced by your arthritis and that the brain picks up on the stimuli from the massage. Many people find that massage leaves them less stressed and more relaxed even if pain reduction is minimal. Talk to your doctor about the role massage can play in your therapy.

Watching Your Weight

Some experts believe that extreme overweight can *cause* osteoarthritis, especially of the knees. A survey reported in the *New York Times* found that seven out of ten New Year's resolutions had to do with personal health and most of them involved weight. It is important to be as close to your ideal weight range as possible because excess weight adds stress to your joints, especially weight-bearing joints such as the hips and knees. This stress will exacerbate your condition and could lead to increased pain. To reduce the impact that weight gain may have, talk to a health care professional about a nutrition and exercise program that can be tailored for you.

Creating a Well-Balanced Diet

The final verdict isn't in yet on what role diet may play in causing or curing arthritis. However, almost everyone will agree that a healthy diet is important to the person with arthritis or any other inflammatory disorder. You need a well-balanced diet, one that includes all major food groups. This will help maintain a healthy body weight. But pain from arthritis may decrease your appetite or lead you to seek substitute gratification through eating ice cream, cakes, and cookies. Or it may be difficult for you to prepare food because of your arthritis. Achieving a well-balanced diet is easier said than done for people with arthritis and other inflammatory disorders.

There is significant evidence that some individuals may set off their inflammatory response by being allergic to certain foods. More and more research is coming out on the immune response in the gut to certain foods and how that may influence the inflammatory process.

The Arthritis Foundation recommends seven guidelines for a healthy diet: (1) Eat a variety of foods, (2) maintain your ideal weight, (3) avoid too much fat and cholesterol, (4) avoid too much sugar, (5) eat foods with enough starch, (6) avoid too much sodium, (7) drink alcohol in moderation. In addition to helping those with inflammatory disorders, a healthy diet improves your immune system, helps you tolerate medication better, improves your appearance, helps you preserve your teeth, and keeps your blood pressure and cholesterol levels low.

It's Never Too Late

A ninety-two year-old woman who suffered from painful arthritis had been unable to walk without assistance for thirty-five years. But at her advanced age, she started an exercise program designed for the elderly. She began exercising at a low level, only gradually increasing her activity. In just six weeks she had improved her condition so much that she was able to go out of the house on her own. This was a woman who had not walked without assistance in thirty-five years! She continued her exercise program and, astoundingly, at the age of ninety-seven, traveled from the United States to London to participate in a walking tour!

If a ninety-two year-old woman with painful arthritis could make such dramatic improvements, think what improvements exercise may bring to you! As research from around the world shows, it's never too late to benefit from exercise. Even the smallest steps can lead to big health benefits.

Learn Self-Management Techniques

Arthritis and the resulting pain and discomfort can be effectively managed. And you can be that manager! If you want to be an effective self-manager: (1) Set long-term goals, such as, "I want to be able to walk up the stairs to my apartment"; (2) determine what you need to do to accomplish your goals; (3) make short-term plans to achieve your goals, such as, "I'm going to add one step each day"; (4) do it—put your plans into action; (5) check your results; (6) modify your plans as needed. There is no promise of a quick cure. But you will see gradual progress if you develop self-management techniques for handling your pain. Those who become effective self-managers experience less pain and live more active lives than those who do not.

Try Talking to Yourself

How we think about things determines how we feel and what we do about problems like pain. How you think about your arthritis pain can affect every aspect of your illness, from the pain itself to your prognosis. Exciting new research shows that you can change the way you think and that changing how you think changes how you behave. To help yourself change the way you talk to yourself, write down any negative thoughts you have about your pain. Next, write those negative thoughts in a positive way. For example, "I'm so stiff and sore I don't want to get out of bed!" can be transformed into, "If I take a nice hot shower or bath, I won't feel so stiff." Positive "self-talk" requires practice. But it can be fun and will make a difference in how you see things and how you behave.

Prevent Pain in the Workplace

You probably spend at least eight hours a day at work, so it is important to make all necessary adjustments to prevent pain from interfering with your job performance. Make sure your chair is properly adjusted so that your arms rest correctly. Your feet should be flat on the floor, with your back straight or supported at a 15- to 20-degree angle. Your desk should be high enough to allow your elbows to rest comfortably. You may want a slanted desktop. This will ease any neck and upper-back strain.

Also, organize your work to save yourself steps and minimize twisting, stooping, or bending. Use equipment that reduces pressure on your joints (e.g., electric stapler, book holders). It is important to change your position every twenty to thirty minutes if you do repetitive work. And if you stand for a long time, raise up one foot occasionally on a stool to rest your back. You can get more specific information by asking your doctor for a referral to an occupational therapist for other tips and ideas geared to your situation.

Reduce Your Stress Levels

Stress is the body and mind's reaction to the pressures and tensions of everyday living. It increases muscle tension and can increase arthritis pain. Stress management is an important part of arthritis treatment. How can you reduce stress levels? By identifying what causes stress in your life; by sharing your thoughts and feelings with someone you trust; by being good to yourself when you are in pain; by simplifying your life as much as possible; by learning to manage your time and conserve your energy; by setting short-term goals for yourself; and by avoiding "solutions" like drugs and alcohol. Available pain and medical support and education services can help you learn how to stay physically and mentally fit.

Go to the Experts

A survey of 1,051 people with arthritis, conducted by the authors of *Arthritis: What Works*, found that most patients consulted at least two or three physicians about their arthritis. Some saw as many as ten doctors. The survey results revealed that rheumatologists and orthopedists were highly recommended for diagnosis and ongoing care; general or family practitioners, osteopaths, and internists were recommended for continuing care; and neurologists were not recommended. The following were recommended for special care: orthopedists for most types of joint surgery, neurosurgeons for neck or back surgery, physiatrists or osteopaths for exercise advice, and rheumatologists for rheumatoid arthritis.

The results also showed that occupational therapists are a tremendous help to people with arthritis. Physical therapists and exercise instructors were the most highly recommended non-M.D. practitioners. Nurses, mental health practitioners, occupational therapists, nutritionists, and dietitians were also highly recommended. Their patients tend to stay active and independent. Nutritionists and dietitians seem the most beneficial to people who seek *and then follow* their advice.

There's Nothing Like a Good Night's Sleep

Good sleep is extremely important for people with inflammatory disorders. Although it has long been known that a good night's sleep is "useful," doctors now consider it *essential.* Many people with arthritis pain develop poor sleep habits and their lack of sleep causes fatigue, which increases pain. The increased pain further disturbs sleep. If you are sleeping poorly, tell your doctor. You may need to adjust your medication to control your pain more effectively. Or you may want to learn some of the valuable relaxation techniques and tips that can help improve your quality of sleep. Don't self-medicate with over-the-counter products, a friend's sleeping pills, or alcohol. Work with your doctor or other practitioner to solve the problem.

Biofeedback

Biofeedback is an effective tool that you can use to learn your unique response to both pain and stress. Biofeedback equipment measures your heart rate, blood pressure, skin temperature, and muscle tension. All of these are indicators of how relaxed or tense you are. Biofeedback can help you monitor how you are really feeling. Often, people with chronic pain think they are relaxed when they are not. Biofeedback provides objective evidence of what is really going on.

Biofeedback itself is not a therapy for pain. It is a way to monitor the effectiveness of other pain-control and relaxation techniques you are using. You will probably need about twelve biofeedback sessions with a specialist (once or twice a week for one hour each session). At home, following the instructions of the biofeedback professional, you can take your own pulse, use an ordinary mirror to see muscles relax, and a use a low-cost ring thermometer to measure body temperature. Generally, people follow an instructional audiotape to help them continue biofeedback on their own. This technique can help you monitor your own progress and control your own pain.

Acupuncture

This ancient technique has value for many problems, and can help with pain control. Practiced in China since at least 3000 B.C.E., acupuncture is becoming increasingly popular in the United States. You may find acupuncture helpful in relieving your pain. Ask your doctor or therapist to recommend a qualified acupuncturist.

In acupuncture, thin needles are inserted at precise points in the body. The procedure can provide relief from pain and even produce anesthesia for certain kinds of surgery. Laser acupuncture (for head and neck pain) and electro-acupuncture (for intense analgesia) are modern modifications of this technique. Acupuncture is safe and effective, with few adverse side effects.

The acupuncture needles stimulate the nerves to block pain signals, and this produces relief from moderate pain for many people. During an acupuncture session, you may feel a slight tingling and/or a warm sensation in your body. Investigators have found that acupuncture improves circulation (poor circulation increases pain), relieves muscle tension (tension increases pain), and stimulates the production of endorphins (the body's natural painkillers) in the brain and spinal cord.

Hypnosis and Self-Hypnosis

In ancient Greece, hypnotic "trances" played a major role in medicine. In the 1800s Franz Mesmer revived interest in hypnotism and healing. And in the early 1900s Sigmund Freud used hypnosis to explore the human mind. There is now renewed interest in hypnosis among physicians, psychiatrists, psychologists, social workers, counselors, and other health professionals. It is an accepted therapeutic technique for managing pain. However, it is not a miracle cure.

Hypnotism is a form of deep relaxation during which your attention is focused inward. Only you can open the door to your unconscious; the hypnotist simply assists you. You may find it helpful to learn self-hypnosis from a trained hypnotist. If you do, you will possess a powerful tool to help you control even severe chronic pain. You can train yourself to enter deep trances and use them therapeutically. Hypnotic suggestions made in self-induced trances can be potent painkillers. You may want to use a prerecorded "induction" tape to help you in and out of trances, especially in the beginning. Tapes are available commercially. Or you may want to make your tape with the help of your hypnotist. Many people discover that hypnosis relieves pain and is a soothing and enjoyable experience on its own as well.

Heat and Cold

What should you choose for pain relief? A hot pack or a cold pack? You may not need to choose between them at all. Both heat and cold are effective in reducing swelling from injury and both help break the pain-spasm-pain cycle that eventually leads to immobility. Heat and cold decrease the number of nerve impulses from the painful area to the spinal cord. You have to find out for yourself which one works best for you under what circumstances.

No matter which you choose, tell your doctor and follow his or her advice, especially with heat treatment. Be sure to put a towel between your skin and whatever type of pack you choose. Hot packs are generally used for no more than twenty minutes under six to eight layers of towels. Cold packs are used for no more than twenty minutes under two layers of towels. If you choose to rub the painful area with ice, do so for no more than ten minutes, or until numbness occurs. Wait until your skin returns to normal temperature (at least twenty minutes) before another application of either heat or cold. Sometimes you may want to try a contrast treatment (i.e., using both heat and cold in combination). First soak the affected area in warm water, then cold water, and then warm water again.

Do not use hot or cold packs if you have open cuts, sores, poor circulation, or vasculitis. Be careful not to use temperatures that are too hot or too cold. And don't use creams, heat rubs, or lotions with hot or cold treatments.

Progressive Muscle Relaxation (PMR)

PMR was developed in the 1930s by Edmund Jacobson and can be of great help in controlling your pain, especially when used in conjunction with biofeedback. Two excellent sources of information on PMR are *The Relaxation and Stress Reduction Workbook* and *The Relaxation Training Program*, both by Thomas Budzynski.

With PMR, you will work with four muscle groups: (1) hands, forearms, and biceps; (2) feet, calves, thighs, buttocks; (3) chest, stomach, and lower back; and (4) shoulders, neck, throat, face, and head. For the best results, do PMR for twenty minutes a day, spending two or three days on each muscle group.

Start by relaxing in a comfortable chair or lying down. Breathe deeply, exhaling slowly. When you are breathing naturally, tense the first muscle group on one side. Hold the muscles tense until you feel a slight burning sensation or cramping (about ten seconds). Relax and feel the muscles in your hands, forearms, and biceps become limp. Repeat this procedure twice, focusing on how your muscles feel. Do one side, then the other. After two or three days, move on to the second muscle group, then the third, and finally the fourth.

PMR is an effective way for you to feel how tense you really are and to let go of that tension. As you relax and become less tense, your pain will diminish as well. If you feel any pain when starting out, go slowly. Avoid overtensing any of the muscle groups.

Twelve Steps for Chronic Pain

Dr. Richard A. Sternbach, director of the Pain Treatment Center at the Scripps Clinic and Research Foundation, has devised a comprehensive, easy-to-follow program that can give you control over your pain. Using the popular "12 Steps" model pioneered by Alcoholics Anonymous and adapted by many other organizations, Dr. Sternbach has synopsized his program into twelve steps for coping with chronic pain.*

1. Accept your pain.
2. Use work, hobbies, and recreation to distract yourself from your pain.
3. Get angry at your pain.
4. Take medications as prescribed.
5. Get fit and stay fit.
6. Use relaxation techniques.
7. Keep active.
8. Pace yourself.
9. Ask for help from family and friends.
10. Be open and honest with your doctor.
11. Share your experiences with others in pain.
12. Stay hopeful.

What to Look For in a Pain Clinic

There are more than 1,000 pain clinics in the United States offering a wide variety of services to the person in pain. With so many pain clinics to choose from, how will you be able to distinguish a high-quality clinic from an average one? Which of the following therapies do you think should be available at a high-caliber pain clinic?

---

* *Adapted from* Mastering Pain: A Twelve-Step Program for Coping with Chronic Pain *(Ballantine Books, 1988), by Dr. Richard A. Sternbach.*

- Trigger point injections
- Nerve blocks
- TENS
- Acupuncture
- Biofeedback
- Total relaxation training
- Self-hypnosis training
- Guided imagery training
- Physical therapy
- Movement therapy
- Individualized exercise programs
- Assertiveness training
- Behavior modification
- Group therapy

Which offerings did you choose? Did you leave any out? All of the therapies listed above should be available at a comprehensive pain clinic. Ask your physician or pain specialist to recommend a clinic if you are interested in investigating the services of a pain center.

Massage for Foot Pain

Every year, you probably walk about 2,000 miles. In a lifetime, most of us walk enough to circle the globe four times. And you wonder why your feet are sore? Pain from sore, aching feet tops the list of common foot complaints. Luckily, many foot problems can be easily self-treated, and pain is one of them. Massaging your feet can bring quick and effective pain relief. Here's one way to massage away your pain:

1. While barefoot, sit in a comfortable chair and put your right foot on your left thigh. Rub your foot with a massage lotion or oil. Using both thumbs, apply pressure to the sole of your foot.
2. Now, make a fist and move your knuckles along the sole of your foot from heel to toe. Do this five times.
3. Next, massage each toe individually. Hold the toe firmly between your thumb and index finger and move it from side to side.

4. Finally, hold all your toes with your right hand and bend them backwards for five to ten seconds. (Steady your foot by holding it with your left hand.)

Do this three times. Repeat the above procedure with your left foot.

Pets Help Relieve Pain

Not everyone wants or is able to keep pets, but they can bring great health benefits, among them pain relief. About 50 percent of physicians and psychologists in the United States recommend that their patients have pets. According to a great deal of reliable research, caring for a pet leads to lower heart rate, blood pressure, and stress levels. Pets also help fight loneliness and depression. And each of these factors is intimately connected with pain intensity.

Pets help you relax. In fact, the act of petting alone lowers blood pressure in many people. The antics of a beloved pet can make you laugh—and laughter is great pain medicine. Pets shift your attention away from yourself, thereby distracting you from your pain, fear, or negative thinking. Dogs and cats top the list of suggested pets, but birds, fish, hamsters, and other animals all fill the bill. According to the editors of *Prevention* magazine, the following are among the "pluses" of having a pet:

- They provide unconditional love and loyal companionship.
- They distract you from your pain and worries.
- They are pleasurable to watch and care for.
- They bring you out of yourself and provide pleasurable activity.
- They—especially dogs—help you get involved in outdoor activities and make it easier to meet people and socialize.
- They make you feel safe.
- They offer constancy in an ever-changing world.
- Petting and touching are physically and emotionally comforting.

Change Your Way of Thinking

How new is mind-body medicine? Chinese physicians knew the mind and body were intimately connected 4,000 years ago. The ancient Greek physicians Hippocrates and Galen knew that thoughts and feelings influence health. Today we know that our thoughts and feelings affect our overall health and perception of pain. But which thoughts and feelings have what effects? Below are some of the major factors that have positive or negative influences on your health, including pain perception.

Positive Influences	love, intimacy, trust, friendship, optimism, altruism, confidence, sense of community, responsibility
Negative Influences	anger, withdrawal, suspicion, fear, pessimism, paranoia, opposition, boredom, feelings of betrayal or of being a victim.

Through psychological techniques such as cognitive therapy, you can learn which types of thoughts most characterize your thinking and *you can learn to change how you think about things*. Negative thoughts will give way to positive ones; pessimism will yield to optimism. You can learn how to strengthen the positive side of yourself. By doing so, you will improve your overall health and even be better able to control your pain.

How can you do this? A good start would be reading *Learned Optimism*, by Martin P. Seligman, Ph.D. It is an excellent guide that will help you to identify how you think and teach you how to change your ways of thinking.

Acupressure

Acupressure is an alternative to acupuncture. It is a procedure you can perform on your own whenever you need quick and effective pain relief. You use your fingers instead of acupuncture needles to affect the acupuncture points, which lie just below the surface of the skin. Researchers believe that both acupuncture and acupressure stimulate the body to produce endorphins—natural painkillers that are 200 times as powerful as morphine.

You will need patience to learn the various pressure points that are connected with different parts of the body. The connections are not always obvious. For example, to relieve back pain, you may need to apply pressure to an acupuncture point on the inside of your thigh. When you become comfortable with this valuable technique, you will be able to use it as needed wherever you may be—at home, on the job, at the mall, or in an uncomfortable airplane seat eight miles up.

Ask your doctor or therapist to recommend a licensed or credentialed acupuncturist who can teach you this technique. Or go to your local library or bookstore and borrow or purchase one of the many excellent guides to acupressure that are available. With acupressure, you can use an ancient technique to help reduce your pain today.

Make Your Own Relaxation Tapes

Although many excellent commercial tapes are available to assist you in relaxation and pain-relief exercises, you may benefit more from a tape you make yourself. You will probably even benefit from making the tape itself. Some people find that they use the relaxation tapes they make for themselves more often than the ones they purchase in a store. This may be because personalized tapes can be made to fit your specific pain needs and living situation.

The "script" for your tape should include the following three elements: (1) breathing, (2) autogenic or self-created phrases, and (3) progressive muscle relaxation. Before you begin taping, sit in a comfortable chair and relax as much as possible. Notice your temperature and how you are breathing. Get a sense of how relaxed you are as you are about to begin. Focus on your breathing at first—you want deep "belly" breathing, not shallow breathing from the chest. When you feel safe and relaxed, begin to repeat your autogenic phrase to yourself (e.g., "My arms and legs are heavy and warm. . .") until your limbs begin to feel heavy and warm. Alternately tighten and relax the muscles in your arms and legs. You will feel your tensions melt away, to be replaced by a pleasurable feeling. Repeat this procedure with all the muscle groups until you are completely relaxed.

For more specific information on making your own tapes to guide you through your relaxation exercises, consult *The Chronic Pain Control Workbook* or any of the many excellent books on this topic.

What to Ask at a Pain Clinic

If you decide to go to a pain clinic because of your chronic pain, you will be asked many questions. Your answers will determine whether or not you are accepted into the pain program. In addition to answering questions put to you by the staff, it is important that you get answers from the staff as well.

Richard M. Linchintz, M.D., author of *Life Without Pain*, suggests that you put the following questions to the staff of the pain clinic. Their answers will help you determine whether you want to be part of their program.

1. What pain specialists are on your staff? Does your program have physical medicine and rehabilitation? Physical therapists? Exercise physiologists? Psychiatrists or psychologists?
2. Does your staff function effectively as a team?
3. What equipment is available (e.g., biofeedback, exercise, physical therapy machines)?
4. Before treatment, do patients receive a comprehensive physical and psychological evaluation? How will the results be used?
5. What subjective factors help determine whether or not a patient is accepted into the program?
6. Does the treatment team tailor individualized programs for patients?
7. Will the team work closely with a patient's doctor?
8. Does the staff work with the patient and his or her family on changing their attitudes toward pain?

It is just as important for you to know if the pain clinic is the right one for you as it is for the staff to know if you are the right patient for their program.

Helping and Healing

In the midst of pain, wouldn't you love to feel a rush of warmth, good feeling, and extra energy? What wouldn't you give for a sense of well-being and self-worth? Well, it turns out that the only thing you may have to give is something that only you have—*yourself!*

Giving to others brings on one of the few "syndromes" you would actually want to have, the "healthy-helping syndrome." Many studies have shown that people who reach out altruistically to help others cope better with chronic pain and other stress-related disorders. They also experience greater overall health and well-being. They experience the so-called "helper's high."

In *The Healing Power of Doing Good: The Health and Spiritual Benefits of Helping Others* by Allan Luks and Peggy Payne, the authors provide exciting information about how helping others helps you. The book also contains a fifty-page guide to over seventy-five national organizations devoted to helping others. Many of these groups could use your help as a volunteer with their work.

According to Luks and Payne, helping can lead to healing if you: (1) have personal contact with those you help, (2) help frequently, (3) help strangers, and (4) help altruistically, without concern for the results or for rewards. You may find pain relief in helping, in giving until it stops hurting.

Reduce Your Pain—Cold Turkey

Research shows that smokers experience twice as much pain as do nonsmokers. One study demonstrated that more than half of all patients with chronic back pain were smokers and 57 percent of those patients needed to smoke more when they were experiencing pain. In addition, people who smoke are usually more reliant on pain medication than nonsmokers. They are also less able to tolerate their pain than nonsmokers.

Since the Surgeon General's Report in 1964, over 30 million Americans have quit smoking. The overwhelming majority of them did it on their own. If you want to quit smoking, the odds are in your favor. No matter why you smoke—because you are "hooked," smoke for "the pleasure of smoking," smoke when you are nervous or under pressure, or because you are psychologically addicted to smoking—quitting smoking will provide two immediate and long-lasting benefits. First, you will feel more energetic within days. Second, you will find that you experience less pain than you did when smoking.

You can do it alone and quit "cold turkey" or you can get the help and advice of your doctor, family, and friends who have quit smoking, or national health organizations that sponsor quit-smoking programs (e.g., American Cancer Society, American Heart Association, American Lung Association). Quitting smoking may be the single best thing you do to improve your health and reduce your pain.

The Benefits of Falling Temperatures

Night pain will prevent you from experiencing the deep, restful sleep that you need. And a lack of "quality sleep" increases the pain that you feel during the day. Few things are as excruciating as lying in bed, unable to sleep, tormented by pain. But there is something you can do about it.

Sleep deepens when your body temperature falls. As your body temperature rises—usually after about five A.M.—you begin to awaken. You can help your body along with this natural process. About two hours before your bedtime, treat yourself to a nice hot bath. Make sure that the bath is very hot—103 degrees Fahrenheit would be perfect.

When you get out of the bath, crawl under the covers immediately, snuggling into bed with your partner (or at least with a good book). You will feel relaxed as your body temperature begins to fall lower and lower. And as your body temperature falls, you will drift into a deeper and deeper sleep. This simple technique can help prevent or break the pain-insomnia-pain cycle and bring you welcome relief during the night and throughout the following day.

Red Hot Chili Peppers for Pain Relief

Since 1991 Americans have bought more salsa than catsup. It may not be too long before another "hot" Mexican food becomes a big seller. You probably know that some foods can cause pain, but do you know that one food relieves pain? In the 1600s, Montezuma put it in a hot chocolate drink. In the 1800s Irish doctors used it to relieve tooth pain. Today, it is being used to control pain from rheumatoid arthritis and osteoarthritis, as well as pain from skin conditions such as herpes zoster and diabetic neuropathy. What is it? Hot chili peppers!

Capsaicin is the ingredient in hot chili peppers that fights pain. It is now widely available and has been proved effective as a pain reliever. Researchers think that capsaicin blocks pain by depleting one of the chemicals the body needs to transmit pain signals to the brain. In a recent study of about 100 patients, capsaicin cream—sold as Zostrix—reduced pain in 57 percent of the patients. Participants in the study found that walking, driving, sitting, and other daily tasks were performed more easily. Also, patients were able to perform exercise regularly as a result of using capsaicin cream—and exercise itself can be an effective therapy for pain relief.

Drugs—When to "Just Say Yes"

Each week nearly 100 million Americans take drugs—medications, that is. And each year Americans spend over $100 billion on drugs to relieve either acute or chronic pain. Painkillers can be divided into two main groups: non-narcotics and narcotics. Both kinds of medication have an important role in relieving pain.

Non-narcotics, such as acetaminophen, aspirin, and ibuprofen, are safe and can be very effective in relieving your pain. In particular, they can help with severe short-term pain. These drugs act on the peripheral nerves; they do not have much effect on the brain directly. They usually come in tablet form and are best taken with liquids and *not* on an empty stomach. A major benefit of the non-narcotics is that they are not addictive. However, these agents should be considered step two in managing chronic pain after natural options and other tactics have been exhausted. If you can combine the use of a natural product with other beneficial activities, you will reduce your need for drug therapy. In this manner, you can achieve substantial benefits over time without risking the harm from the side effect of drugs.

Narcotics, such as morphine and related drugs, are far more powerful than the non-narcotics. They slow or stop the pain signals that are processed by the central nervous system. When properly used, narcotic drugs allow people in pain to lead normal lives. Although these drugs can be addictive, most people do not get "hooked" and have no trouble stopping when the drug is no longer needed. However, withdrawal symptoms from the drug may cause some difficulty and the pain may increase for a brief period after discontinuing the drug. When you are in pain and a drug is suggested to control or reduce that pain, the best response may be to just say yes.

It's The Real Thing—Placebo!

Many years ago, in his opening monologue on *Saturday Night Live*, the comedian Steve Martin recommended that everyone in the audience take the drug he had taken just before coming on stage. "It's called *place-bo*," he said, mispronouncing the word. A placebo is a remedy that has no direct effect on the disease. It may be a just sugar pill or an injection of saltwater. However, up to 90 percent of patients get some pain relief after taking a placebo. Even though they are not "real" drugs, placebos are powerful medicine.

Endorphins—the body's natural opiates—seem to play a role in the effectiveness of placebos. In one study of twenty-three dental patients who had teeth extracted, researchers found that 33 percent of the subjects experienced pain relief after being injected with a placebo. When those individuals were injected with a drug that blocked endorphins, their pain returned, suggesting that the patient's belief in the placebo led to the production of painkilling endorphins.

The effectiveness of the placebo indicates that we have within us self-regulatory, self-healing capacities that can be harnessed to bring about healing. Although the placebo may not be considered "the real thing," it appears to mobilize the real healing process within us. Perhaps Hippocrates had it right thousands of years ago when he said, "The natural healing force within each one of us is the greatest force in getting well."

There is a catch-22 involved in using a placebo to control pain: you cannot know it is a placebo. It seems that believing that someone or something is helping to relieve your pain is essential at times to having that pain relieved.

Therapeutic Touch

Is therapeutic touch for you? Could it help relieve your pain? You may want to do some reading on the subject or attend a lecture in your area. Many schools now offer accredited courses on the subject. And many hospitals have practitioners of this modality on their staffs. Dolores Krieger, Ph.D., a professor of nursing at New York University, is one of the contemporary pioneers in therapeutic touch. She is the author of a book on the subject—*Therapeutic Touch*—and tours the country giving workshops. Barbara Brennan, author of *Hands of Light*, is another respected expert practitioner of this ancient art.

How does therapeutic touch work? The whole story is not completely understood yet, but it seems that a *transfer of energy* is involved from one person to the other. Body temperature plays a key role. Healers search out an area of temperature change in the body and then perform a "laying on of the hands" over the affected area. Deep heat is usually felt at these times. The healer does not need to actually touch the area to be effective.

Are the effects of this technique simply the results of the power of suggestion? Research suggests that more is going on—healers have influenced the growth of plants and seeds. And hemoglobin levels are higher in patients treated with therapeutic touch compared with patients not so treated. Research so far indicates that something real is happening, but we don't yet know what it is.

The skin is the largest organ in the body. It is essential to our survival. We also perceive and express love through the skin and touch—mothers keep their babies close, lovers hold one another, parting friends hug good-bye. And it is through the skin, through therapeutic touch, that some are able to transfer that most powerful force that heals the sick—*love*.

Cutting Out Caffeine

You may be addicted to the most widely used drug in the world and inadvertently increasing the pain that you feel. Are you addicted to gaweh without knowing it? Perhaps you know it as kahveh or kaffee or—coffee.

The jolt that you get from coffee, many sodas, or over-the-counter "medicines" is caused by caffeine. The caffeine from coffee hits about thirty minutes after your first sip and lasts from two to eight hours after the last good drop. Caffeine raises your blood sugar rapidly and that brings you up.

However, it also causes a rise in your insulin levels—and that eventually brings you down. Too much caffeine overstimulates the nervous system and causes the "jitters."

More than 300 mg of caffeine a day can cause increased heart rate, increased blood pressure, insomnia, nervousness, and irritability—all of which are associated with pain. You get 300 mg of caffeine in three six-ounce cups of coffee, six cups of tea, or six cans of soda. And some popular over-the-counter products have as much as 200 mg of caffeine in each pill. Some common pain relievers have from 30 to 65 mg of caffeine in each tablet.

Cutting out coffee will help you reduce your pain by stopping the overstimulation of your central nervous system. Many people choose to taper off coffee and cut out one or two cups each week. Some people substitute herbal teas for their morning coffee or drink coffee substitutes like chicory or the roasted ground beans of barley, wheat, or chestnut. Others just switch to decaf. You may want to use one of the many popular relaxation techniques available to help you cut out caffeine. These techniques can also help you learn to relax and fill the role once played by a satisfying cup of coffee.

Massaging with Topical Lotions

Massage brings warmth and reduced pain to sore areas because it increases blood flow. Unless you have pain in your shoulders, elbows, wrists, or fingers—from arthritis, for example—you can give yourself a relaxing, pleasurable massage. If you can't practice self-massage, ask your doctor or physical therapist to recommend an experienced, trained professional.

Oils and lotions can increase the relaxing quality of a massage. They make the hands feel as if they are smoothly gliding over your skin. Many people discover that by using menthol gels their pain is further eased. The "tingle" from the menthol does wonders to soothe the painful area. You may also want to try some topical "deep heating" rubs. Some effective topical rubs contain medicines that block pain sensations. Others cause increased blood flow to the skin where they are applied and this helps relieve the pain. In general, topical lotions and ointments do not penetrate deeply into the skin.

If you are massaging yourself, stop as soon as you feel any pain and never massage a swollen or painful joint. If you plan to use a heat treatment after your self-massage, make sure you remove any menthol gel that you may have used. If you don't, you might burn yourself. A good massage will relax you, distract you, and help reduce your pain.

Music and Pain Relief

Would you rather take a pill or play a CD when you are in pain? If you go for the pill, you may have chosen the less effective method. A tape of soothing music may bring you more pain relief at times than medication. Some doctors even *prescribe* twenty minutes of beautiful music for their patients instead of medication. At Kaiser Permanente in Los Angeles, doctors use music to help relieve pain in their patients with chronic pain, back problems, migraine, ulcers, high blood pressure, and other stress-related disorders.

Music is a powerful tool. It can magically transform your mood. Pythagoras had a daily music regimen—he awoke to, worked with, and relaxed to music throughout the day. Ancient physicians used music as part of healing. Today music is often used along with biofeedback and hypnosis to bring pain relief. Music affects the "thinking" part of the brain (cerebral cortex), the "emotional" part (limbic system), and the "primitive" part (brain stem). Some researchers believe that music stimulates the body to produce its own natural painkillers—endorphins.

Music can transport you far away from your pain. Some find just what they need in classical music, others in Broadway show tunes, and still others in rap. At Kaiser Permanente, doctors recommend the harp music of Georgia Kelly. Many people enjoy Kitaro's *Silk Road*, Steve Halpern's *Spectrum Suite*, Diana Keck's visualization sound tapes, *Healing the Emotions* and *Transforming Mental Habits*.

You may find that you enjoy Handel, Brahms, Beethoven, or the Beatles. The music of Vaughan Williams, Debussy, or Eric Satie may be just what you need. Native American flute music—*Canyon Trilogy* by R. Carlos Nakai, for example—or Irish harp music by O'Carolan, "new age" Celtic music by Enya, or the dulcet sounds of James Galway performing music from around the world all may be beautiful aesthetic experiences that also help relieve your pain.

Effective Affirmation

Negative thinking can bring on or exacerbate painful feelings. One way to fight negative thinking is through positive thinking. Positive thinking expressed in the form of daily affirmations is particularly effective. What is an affirmation? It's a positive statement that you can use to change a negative belief or expectation. An affirmation is also a tool to help you move in a new direction. Shakti Gawain's book *Reflections in the Light: Daily Thoughts and*

Affirmations is an excellent collection of affirmations that you can use to trigger your own thoughts and feelings each day.

How do you use affirmations? The one Gawain wrote for the date this is being written is, "I value who I am." A few days ago the affirmation was, "I am sending clear, loving thought messages from my mind to my body." The author suggests you read the affirmation and the commentary that goes with it in the morning, think about it for a while, and—if you like it—write it out a few times. If you don't like the affirmation in the book, write your own! In the evening, reread the affirmation, reflect on your day, and write down your thoughts.

Below are some suggestions for using affirmations effectively:

- Use your favorite relaxation technique to get into the proper state of mind.
- Keep your affirmations simple.
- State your affirmations in the present tense.
- Make your affirmations positive.
- If negative thinking raises its ugly head, stop that train of thought and continue with your positive affirmation.
- Let yourself feel the positive sensations that come with your affirmations.
- Keep your written affirmations with you during the day where you can see them as needed.
- Make positive affirmation a part of your everyday life.

Pain relief is just an affirmation away.

The Human Comedy

The famous comedian Charlie Chaplin once said, "Life is a tragedy when seen in close-up, but a comedy in long shot." And what is true of our lives is also true of our pain. The more you focus on your pain, the worse it feels. The more distractions you put between your self and your pain, the better you feel. In one study, researchers asked dental patients to rate their pain every five minutes. Then they were asked to rate their pain every thirty minutes. Much more pain was reported by the patients who thought about their pain at five-minute intervals than by those who waited thirty minutes before assessing their pain.

Norman Cousins reported in his landmark book, *Anatomy of an Illness*, that watching old movie comedies helped him relieve his pain. Because of

VCRs and DVDs, thousands and thousands of old movies are now readily available at the corner video store or through the mail for those in more remote areas. The classic films of Charlie Chaplin, Buster Keaton, Ben Turpin, Laurel and Hardy, Mack Sennett, and the many other comedy stars of the silent era are available today. The zany comedy of the Marx Brothers, the eccentric humor of W. C. Fields, the sophisticated comedies of Ernst Lubitsch or Preston Sturges are all on tape.

Who makes you laugh the most? Bill Cosby? Eddie Murphy? Bill Murray? Peter Sellers? Jerry Lewis? George Burns? Lucille Ball? Lily Tomlin? Bette Midler? Steve Martin? George Carlin? Mary Tyler Moore? Dick Van Dyke? Bob Newhart? Jerry Seinfeld? Woody Allen? Whoever it is that provokes you to uncontrolled hilarity, you can most certainly find his or her material on videotape or audiotape.

Many people keep a comedy tape by the bedside VCR or cassette recorder and have a good laugh just before sleep or just after waking. A good laugh can help change your focus from the tragic close-up that increases your pain to the comic long shot that you need. "Laugh and be well," Matthew Green wrote in 1737. This is as true today as it was then.

Prayer

From the 23rd Psalm in the Old Testament to the Our Father in the New Testament to the "Jesus Prayer" in J. D. Salinger's *Franny and Zooey*, people the world over have prayed and found relief from pain and suffering through their prayers.

The dictionary defines *prayer* as "a reverent petition made to God, a god or another object of worship . . . a fervent request." For many people of widely divergent religious views, the act of praying is a source of comfort and relaxation.

You may find that listening to a tape of an inspirational message by a religious leader eases your pain. Or you may want to make a tape recording of yourself reading your favorite prayers. You can listen to the tape at home, on your Walkman during a break at work, or in your car. Also, there is a wide range of books of prayer available to meet the religious needs of anyone from Anabaptists to Zen Buddhists, as well as the spiritual needs of theists, agnostics, and even atheists. The value of praying for others regardless of great physical distance has been evaluated and proved scientifically to help the healing process.

Prayer may not be for everyone, but at one time or another it may just work for you.

Pace Yourself

"Slow down you move too fast," Simon and Garfunkel sang. The pace of modern life continues to increase daily. If you experience chronic pain, you—more than most—need to learn how to pace your activities. It is important not to push yourself beyond your limits. You can avoid a lot of pain by learning when to take a quiet break. A few minutes of rest will keep you feeling well and help you stay productive throughout the workday. If you are on a vacation, add time for rest periods throughout the day while touring the countryside or exploring a new city. Don't cram your itinerary with so many events that you wear yourself out.

When exercising, vary your routine so you use different muscle groups. Whether you're at work or involved in a hobby at home, don't spend too much time at any one activity. Get up and move about if you have been sitting for a while; find a comfortable chair and listen to a relaxing tape for a few minutes if you have been on your feet. Learning to pace yourself will help you avoid and reduce pain.

The Alexander Technique

While it is valuable to change ways of thinking and behaving that cause or increase pain, you may also find pain relief in altering your habitual ways of moving. Frederick Alexander developed a technique that can help you accomplish this.

As a young actor Alexander experienced certain problems on stage that led him to study himself carefully. He came to see that how we move affects our total being—physical, emotional, and mental. The Alexander Technique, developed by the young actor, is designed to help you eliminate negative habitual movement patterns. The technique allows you to develop a heightened awareness of the everyday physical habits. Through the Alexander Technique, you learn new, more natural ways of moving that replace your old habits.

The Alexander Technique may help people with bone or muscle pain, osteoarthritis, trigeminal neuralgia, and many other conditions as well. As your old ways of moving are replaced, you may find that headaches, backaches, and many other types of chronic pain vanish along with them. You can learn more about this technique by reading *The Use of Self, the Alexander Technique* by William Barlow, or Edward Maisel's book, also titled *The Alexander Technique.*

The Feldenkrais Technique

This technique of body movement retraining was developed by a physicist, Dr. Moshe Feldenkrais, and involves two separate but related techniques: (1) group-based awareness through movement and (2) private treatment sessions called functional integration.

The Feldenkrais Technique is a system of movement that is designed to eliminate stress and tension from your body, both of which exacerbate pain. In the Feldenkrais system, there are no doctors and patients, only pupils and teachers. The instructor uses extremely gentle touching and muscle manipulation to help you learn to move your muscles in a more natural way. The work on your body may also reduce much of the emotional and mental stress that frequently accompanies tense musculature.

Dr. Feldenkrais has worked with actors, dancers, professional athletes (such as former basketball star Julius Erving), and children with cerebral palsy. If you have a neuromuscular injury or chronic pain—especially back pain—you may want to consider the Feldenkrais Technique. You can learn more about this technique from Dr. Feldenkrais's book *Awareness Through Movement.*

Breaking Pain-Related Habits

How many of your daily habits are intimately connected with the pain you experience? Do you smoke? Drink more than you want to? Get enough exercise? Do you eat right? Whatever the habit is, even if it is difficult to break, you can replace a bad habit with a good habit. Experts say it takes about three weeks to accomplish this. Here are four steps that can help you break pain-related habits.

1. Identify the pain-related habit. Be honest with yourself. Is pain a result of what or how much you eat, your posture, or lack of exercise? Write down the habits that you feel are causing or contributing to your pain.
2. Identify your goals in changing these habits. Do you want to exercise more to become more physically active and have more energy? Do you want to lose weight to be more attractive to your spouse or to relieve your arthritic joints of added pressure? Write down the reasons why you want to change your habits.
3. Identify at least one healthy habit that will replace each pain-related habit you want to change. Instead of watching TV, substitute a brisk forty-five-minute walk three times a week.

Instead of stopping for a beer with the guys after work, join a health club in the neighborhood. Write down the healthy habits you plan to substitute for your pain-related habits.

4. Identify the rewards you will give yourself for successfully following through on your plan to replace pain-related habits with healthy habits. Buy yourself a new Walkman or Discman and tapes or CDs to listen to when you go for your evening walks. Treat yourself to a new outfit, one that accents your improved physical appearance. Write down the many ways you are going to be good to yourself for taking care of yourself to help you maintain your new healthy habits.

Are You Determined?

Dr. David E. Bresler, an expert in pain management, has compared many of his patients to "ships without captains." According to Dr. Bresler, the key to successfully combating your pain is the intensity of your motivation to get better. He arrived at this conclusion based on his work with thousands of patients with pain. The following seven items are needed to achieve the level of motivation that Dr. Bresler thinks are the key to success.

1. Take a good look at yourself and your life.
2. Replace negative attitudes and behavior with positive ones.
3. Explore and learn what's out there to help you with your pain (e.g., acupuncture, meditation, a change in diet), and approach them with an open mind.
4. Experiment and try new ways of controlling or eliminating your pain. Keep what works; let go of what doesn't.
5. Create your own pain-control techniques using what you've learned from others.
6. Prepare yourself for setbacks. They are only temporary and happen to everybody.
7. Always remember: *You have the power* to master your pain.

Glove Anesthesia

William Kroger, M.D., developed this pain-relief technique. With this simple imagery exercise, your hand becomes like an anesthetic glove. It is particularly helpful when intense pain makes it difficult for you to use other meditation or guided imagery techniques that require more concentration and effort. Glove anesthesia can help you to "take the edge off" your pain quickly. The technique also gives you power and control over your pain. The more you practice glove anesthesia, the easier it gets. And the more you use this technique, the longer and longer the pain relief lasts.

First, get comfortable. Then focus on your slow, deep breathing. Close your eyes and imagine that a bucket of clear, potent liquid anesthetic has been placed before you. Dip your hand into the bucket up to your wrist, moving it around and in and out. You will begin to feel a tingly sensation come over your hand as the anesthetic takes effect. The numbness will spread deep into your bones. Then swirl your hand around in the bucket. Now remove your hand from the bucket and touch the part of your body that hurts, allowing the numbness to flow from your hand into that painful area. Dip your hand back into the bucket and repeat the exercise as many times as you like.

You may want to buy a prerecorded audiotape to help you and guide you through this exercise, or make one for yourself. After you have done it a number of times, you will be able to perform the glove anesthesia technique on your own without assistance.

When Medicines + Exercise = Pain

It is important to make regular exercise a part of your life. And there are times when you may need to take medication to treat a medical condition or for pain relief. Usually, neither activity will cause you any problems. However, combining exercise with some medications can be hazardous. Among the medications you should avoid when you are exercising are aspirin, antihistamines, diuretics, and tranquilizers. Why? Aspirin masks pain. You may continue exercising when you should stop, resulting in injury and pain. Antihistamines can lead to strain on the heart and muscles. Diuretics can lead to dehydration and painful cramps. Tranquilizers distort pain perception and may lead to overexercise, causing injury and pain. And the overuse of any medication can lead to pain at any time, not just during exercise. Overuse of drugs can hinder the body's natural pain-fighting capacities.

Vitamins and Pain

The role vitamins play in good health has been increasingly recognized and investigated. Research indicates that vitamins help fight everything from the common cold to certain kinds of cancer. In general, it is safe and beneficial to take vitamins as part of a healthy diet. However, consider getting advice from a qualified professional on what vitamins and minerals you should take, especially if you are curretnly on any medications.

Chinese Herbal Medicine for Pain

In Western medicine the body is viewed as a machine and doctors are "mechanics" who specialize in fixing the various parts that break down. In Chinese medicine, the human body is seen as a garden in which both patient and doctor are "gardeners" who work to restore and maintain harmony with nature. Western medicine works with powerful synthetic chemicals in accordance with its biochemical view of health and disease. Chinese medicine works with potent herbs and other natural substances in accordance with its views of bio-energy, expressed in the opposing energy forces called yin and yang.

A number of the herbal remedies used in Chinese medicine can be effective in treating chronic pain. Whereas Western medications treat the symptoms of a disease, herbal remedies treat the underlying causes. These are determined by diagnosis according to the principles of Chinese medicine, not Western medicine. Unwanted side effects are rare with Chinese herbal medicine.

In Chinese medicine *qi* (pronounced *chee*; the name for the Life Energy), moisture, and blood circulate within the body in pathways called channels. When they flow smoothly, you feel healthy; when their flow is disrupted, illness results and you may feel such symptoms as joint pain, headache, anxiety, fatigue, high blood pressure, menstrual cramps, and the common cold. Herbal remedies regulate the flow of qi, moisture, and blood to restore or maintain health.

Chinese herbs are combined or compounded into formulas that are available in a variety of forms—liquid bottled extracts, ground herbs in pill form, powders, and herbs to be boiled into tea. Herbal remedies can be used for such conditions as arthritis, backache, herpes zoster, high blood pressure, menstrual pain, neuralgia, TMJ, and ulcers. There are some practitioners who feel that commercial preparations are not as effective as remedies made specifically for you by a Chinese herbalist. On the other hand, many formulas have been passed down through traditional Chinese medicine that were developed for a variety of specific conditions. Chinese and Western medicine can be used successfully as complements to one another. If you want to learn more about Chinese medicine in general and herbal remedies in particular, you may want to read *Between Heaven and Earth: A Guide to Chinese Medicine*, by Harriet Beinfield, L.Ac., and Efrem Korngold, L.Ac., O.M.D.; or *The Web That Has No Weaver: Understanding Chinese Medicine*, by Ted J. Kaptchuk, O.M.D. In addition, *Outline Guide to Chinese Herbal Patent Medicines in Pill Form: An Introduction to Chinese Herbal Medicines*, by Margaret A. Naeser, Ph.D., is an excellent resource. Or visit www.Intramedicine.com, which is developing a fully interactive database.

Reflexology

Reflexologists believe that life energy moves through your body in ways yet to be determined. In the 1920s Dr. W. Fitzgerald divided the body into energy zones and developed what is now called reflexology. This technique may not be entirely new. A form of reflexology may have been in use in both ancient Egypt and ancient China. However, in our era it was introduced into the United States by Eunice D. Ingham through her book *Stories the Feet Can Tell*, which was published in 1932. Reflexology involves a gentle stroking of areas of blocked energy or a deep pressure similar to that used in shiatsu. The pressure may cause a slight pain at times. Often sessions begin with breathing exercises to relax the patient.

Reflexology has helped many people with their pain, especially with back pain. It may also help with arthritis, sinus headache, migraine, and hypertension. You can learn more about this technique in *Reflexology for Good Health*, by Anna Kaye and Don C. Matcham.

Osteopathy

Andrew Taylor Still, a Union doctor in the Civil War, founded this school of medicine. Osteopathy is concerned with establishing and maintaining sound body structure, basically through manipulation of the joints and spine. For the osteopath, good health depends on the spine. In the United States today, doctors of osteopathy are recognized, licensed doctors, able to practice and prescribe medication in almost every state. Increasingly, patients are seeing osteopaths for help with their arthritis, sciatica, "tennis elbow," and other inflammatory conditions that are not responding to conventional therapy.

Osteopaths appear to have great success in working with people who have back pain, particularly the kind of lower-back pain that used to be called lumbago. They can also provide help to people who have strained their backs gardening or picking up something incorrectly.

Chiropractic Therapy

For decades the American medical establishment, especially the American Medical Association (AMA), sought to destroy chiropractic medicine in the United States. In 1990 the U.S. Supreme Court put an end to the AMA campaign against this form of medicine when it upheld a lower court ruling that the AMA had engaged in a conspiracy to "contain and eliminate" (those were the AMA's own words) the chiropractic profession. The court found the AMA guilty of antitrust violations and levied a series of penalties against the organization, including substantial fines.

Today chiropractic medicine is recognized by the AMA, allopathic physicians often refer their patients to chiropractors, and the treatment is one of the mainstays for lower-back pain. In the 1980s and 1990s a number of studies were done outside of the United States that demonstrated that after just two to three weeks, between 79 and 93 percent of patients with disabling back pain reported significantly decreased pain and increased mobility. Since then, many studies in the United States and abroad have shown that chiropractic treatment is effective for lower-back pain. Surveys of patients reveal that chiropractors help bring relief for moderate lower-back and neck pain. Gentler forms of manipulation appear to produce better results. Chiropractors who ask about the patient's lifestyle, stress levels, and exercise patterns produce better results than those who do not discuss these topics.

Be Good to Yourself

Don't let pain get in the way of a summer getaway or other vacation. You can visit the most beautiful places on earth, have a fabulous vacation, and in doing so find pain relief and physical rejuvenation.

Many hotels, lodges, and retreats offer "wellness" vacations along with their beautiful locations. These spas are now found even in Las Vegas! You can sign up for different kinds of massage therapy, aromatherapy, hydrotherapy, herbal wraps, whirlpools, saunas, steam rooms, swimming, and hot/cold contrast pools. You have the opportunity to work out on exercise equipment, receive nutritional counseling, learn stress-management techniques, and participate in smoking-cessation and weight-loss classes. You can do any or all of this and engage in all the other activities you enjoy too.

Spas offer special opportunities to pamper your pain away. They have long been meccas for Europeans seeking physical and spiritual renewal, and many excellent luxury spas are in operation in the United States today, from Maine to Hawaii. A good travel agent can help you choose the right place for you and your family. You may also want to read *Spa Finders* magazine or the latest edition of *The Best Spas*, by Theodore B. Van Italie and Leila Hadley. *Healthy Traveler* magazine is another good source of information.

Self-Massage for Neck Pain

There isn't any one technique you can use to massage away your neck pain, but the following general advice should be helpful. Get into bed and relax. Put a small pillow under your head and neck and assume the fetal position. Then put a pillow between your knees as well. Lie down on your left side. Apply oil or a lotion to the right side of your neck, the back of your neck, and your right shoulder with your left hand. Massage directly below your right ear and apply a gentle pressure in small circular motions. Slowly work your way down your neck to your shoulder. Take your time. Massage in a relaxed manner, until you feel you have done as much as you can. When you are done, roll over onto your right side and repeat the procedure. This technique does not provide a panacea for pain but it should help relieve your neck pain.

Osteoarthritis and Back Pain

Physiatrists, physical therapists, and rheumatologists may help you the most if your back pain is caused by osteoarthritis. You may also get pain relief for this condition by working with yoga instructors, physical fitness instructors, or kinesiologists (the last use a technique that assesses nutritional status on the basis of the response of the muscles to mechanical stress). Physical therapy and individualized exercise instruction can also provide much help, as can yoga and tai chi.

However, you can help yourself the most by walking regularly, swimming, performing back exercises daily, reducing stress in your life, using heat therapy when appropriate, getting enough sleep and rest, watching your weight, and using heel cushions in your shoes.

Self-Help Program for Arthritis

The Arthritis Foundation offers a program designed to help patients learn how to reduce pain and maintain normal or near-normal levels of functioning. This self-help program is not a panacea but it does help many people and can even lead to lower medical expenses for some. Nonprofessionals who suffer from arthritis and who have undergone training lead the foundation's program. The program takes a group approach and uses a wide range of techniques such as contracts, goal setting, feedback from group members, and education to help arthritis sufferers. For more information, contact your local office of the Arthritis Foundation.

"Batherapy"

Do you find it difficult or even painful to take a bath because of muscle or nerve pain? For some people, it is hard to relax in the tub because it is difficult for them to lean back or sit up in the bath. The following tips may help you get the most benefit out of your bath.

- Limit your baths to no more than twenty minutes.
- Use warm water rather than hot water.
- Fill the tub as high as possible to take pressure off muscles and nerves.
- When taking a bath, lean against the back of the tub. Raise your knees and keep your feet flat against the bottom of the tub.
- Use an inflatable bath pillow with suction cups that attach to the tub; this will help you lean back more comfortably and take pressure off your neck and back.
- Put a hand towel between the tub and the small of your back for support.

A bath can be a great way to relieve stress, tension, and chronic pain. And these tips will help make your bath more relaxing and effective in reducing pain.

The Healthiest Exercise

It's aerobic, nonweight-bearing, great for stretching, and terrific for strengthening almost all of your muscles. It's one of the best—if not the best—exercise for you to add to your exercise routine. What is it? Swimming!

Most people with chronic pain will discover that swimming reduces their pain. Many people with back pain—even pain from a ruptured disk—find swimming may help ease their pain. In fact, swimming is often considered to be superior to back exercises for pain relief. A large number of people with pain from osteoarthritis find that swimming only fifteen minutes every other day helps relieve their pain. In addition, a number of patients find that swimming is an effective way to handle pain from sciatica and from scoliosis. However, you will probably want to avoid the breaststroke or butterfly stroke if you have any back problems. The overhand crawl is not recommended for people with chronic pain. The sidestroke is easiest if you have back pain. When you swim, make sure there is a lifeguard on duty. Also, use goggles to protect your eyes, and take a hot shower or hot bath when you are finished.

Why Didn't Anyone Tell Me about Myotherapy?

Bonnie Prudden, a leading authority on physical fitness and exercise therapy, who helped President Eisenhower create the President's Council on Physical Fitness, devised a pain-relief technique that she calls myotherapy. According to Prudden, 95 percent of all pain originates in the muscles. Her technique—Pain Erasure—focuses on "trigger points" in muscles. These points are caused by "insult" or damage to the muscles. In some cases, she believes, this damage can be caused *in utero*.

Frequently these trigger points remain dormant for decades. Later in life, when they are activated by emotional or physical stress, they cause various kinds of pain. With myotherapy, you can erase the pain by applying pressure to your muscles using your fingers, knuckles, and elbows. Myotherapy can help with arthritis and bursitis, "tennis elbow," tension headaches, jaw pain, lower-back pain, shin splints, and other conditions.

To learn more about this technique and how it may help you, pick up a copy of *Pain Erasure, the Bonnie Prudden Way*, by Bonnie Prudden. This how-to book explains the theory behind the technique and gives the reader practical, illustrated examples of specific techniques that can be used to get relief from your pain.

The Bethesda Pain Control Program

Bruce Smoller, M.D., and Brian Schulman, M.D., the founders of the Bethesda Pain Control Program, have shown that anyone can learn to reduce and control his or her pain. Their program aims at helping you become an "educated consumer" and an active participant in your own health care. Trained in medicine, orthopedics, and psychiatry, these two doctors have devised a pain-control program with this guiding principle: *You are responsible for the control of your pain.*

The first part of their three-part program involves educating you to understand the nature and mechanisms of pain and the potential pain control offered by various treatments. The second part helps you understand the impact pain is having on your daily life. And the third part involves your coming to see that much of your pain is what they call a "learned maladaptive behavior."

By the end of the program, you will have learned how to create your own pain-control program. These physicians also believe that keeping a personal record—a pain diary—is essential to your success in controlling your pain. The Bethesda Pain Control Program does not replace any other work you may be doing with your physician, therapist, or on your own. It complements it. You can learn more about this program by reading *Pain Control: The Bethesda Program*, by Bruce Smoller, M.D., and Brian Schulman, M.D.

Pain Control without Drugs

Neal H. Olshan, Ph.D., has created a fourteen-day pain-control program. Dr. Olshan devised his plan in an attempt to control his own pain. It worked for him and he believes it can help you control your pain. Dr. Olshan's program does not involve any of what he calls "the four Ms"—magic words, miracle cures, mysterious pills, or marvelous promise. What is the key to this program? It causes the body to produce its own natural painkillers—the endorphins.

His program can be done anywhere. No surgery or medication is involved and it is compatible with any medical care you are receiving. It doesn't disrupt your daily routine. Dr. Olshan does not promise that you will be completely pain-free within two weeks. However, he says his program will bring some relief in fourteen days. Pain relief will increase the longer you practice the plan. His pain-control program can help with arthritis and other inflammatory conditions, back pain, neuralgias, sciatica, muscle pain, neck pain, and headaches. To learn more about this approach, read *Power Over Your Pain Without Drugs: Dr. Olshan's 14-Day Pain Control Program*, by Neal H. Olshan, Ph.D.

Walk That Pain Right Out of Your Life

Walking strengthens the heart, lungs, muscles, and bones. It relieves tension and makes you feel more energetic. Walking is easy for most people. It doesn't cost anything and it's safe. You can walk alone when you need time by yourself or you can walk with friends when you need company. Walking can lead you to many beautiful experiences. For example, walk through a nearby park or along the banks of a river and enjoy the early morning or evening. Go for a long walk at sunset along the beach, feel the sea wind at your back, and savor the salty sea air.

Or your walk may take you to a museum filled with art treasures, ancient artifacts, or scientific wonders. You may walk through the streets of your hometown or city on a guided or self-guided tour, looking with new eyes at familiar buildings and locales of historic interest. Both the walking and the things you see and do will help reduce your pain.

A flat, level route is generally best for those in pain because it minimizes stress on the hips, knees, and feet. Remember to warm up before you go for a brisk walk and to "cool down" at the end with a stroll. Pace yourself. It takes practice to find the walking speed that is right for you. Good shoes are essential. They don't have to be expensive but they do need to be the proper size, with shock-absorbing soles and insoles. A shoe with a cork, continuous crepe, or composite sole is best.

Create Your Own Pain–Control Smorgasbord

Some years ago Dr. Bob Arnot—the TV doctor for CBS—put together an excellent series called "Stop the Pain." Dr. Arnot looked at what people were doing around the country to fight their pain: a headache clinic in Cleveland, a "regular" doctor in New York City working full time with a Chinese acupuncturist/herbalist, water therapy for elderly patients, biomagnetic therapy, a transdermal patch system, a spinal stimulator, an implantable pump, new drugs for migraine, chemotherapy for arthritis, and other methods. Dr. Arnot put together a lot of useful information.

But you don't have to be a TV doctor to collect information. You can do the same thing and find what you can use to get relief from your pain. Bookstores and libraries are filled with valuable books and tapes. Some medical libraries in your area may be open to the public. They have professional journals devoted to pain and pain relief. In addition, there are good Web sites available. Daily newspapers, weekly or monthly magazines, and TV and radio shows often feature stories on the work being done by researchers and physicians in the field of pain control. Many excellent consumer-oriented health newsletters are available that can keep you up to date about exciting advances in treating pain.

Create your own library of information—print, videotape, and audio-tape—on pain and pain control. In your library you will have valuable information that will help you control your own pain. You can create a smorgasbord of pain-control techniques from which you can pick and choose as needed. You may soon find that you have twenty-four-hour access to the best pain-control expert around—you!

Resources

BOOKS

Most of the following books can be found on the Internet or at your local bookstore. If not, ask your bookstore to order them.

General

Benjamin, Ben, and Gail Borden. *Listen to Your Pain*, New York: Viking, 1984.

Chodron, Pema. *When Things Fall Apart: Heart Advice for Difficult Times*. Boston: Shambhala, 1997.

Cohen, Darlene. *Finding a Joyful Life in the Heart of Pain*. Boston: Shambhala, 2000.

Cousins, Norman. *Anatomy of an Illness as Perceived by the Patient*. New York: Bantam Doubleday Dell, 1991.

Dychtwald, Ken. *Bodymind*. Los Angeles: Jeremy P. Tarcher, 1986.

Egoscue, Pete. *Pain-Free: A Revolutionary Method for Stopping Chronic Pain*. New York: Bantam Doubleday Dell, 2000.

Gawain, Shakti. *Creative Visualization*. Novato, Calif.: New World Library, 1995.

Hay, Louise. *You Can Heal Your Life*. Carlsbad, Calif.: Hay House, 1999.

Kabat-Zinn, Jon. *Full Catastrophe Living: Using the Wisdom of Your Body and Mind to Face Stress, Pain, and Illness*. McHenry, Ill.: Delta, 1990.

Laskow, Leonard. *Healing with Love: A Breakthrough Mind-Body Medical Program for Healing Yourself and Others*. Wholeness Press, 1992.

Lewis, C. S., *The Problem of Pain*. Carmichael, Calif.: Touchstone Books, June 1996.

Siegel, Bernie S. *Love, Medicine and Miracles*. New York: Harper Perennial, 1990.

Zand, Janet, Allen Spreen, and James LaValle. *Smart Medicine for Healthier Living*. New York: Avery Publishing, 1999.

Arthritis

Horstman, Judith, et al. *The Arthritis Foundation's Guide to Alternative Therapies.* Marietta, Ga.: Longstreet Press, 1999.

Newmark, Thomas, and Paul Schulick. *Beyond Aspirin: Nature's Challenge to Arthritis, Cancer and Alzheimer's Disease.* Prescott, Ariz.: Hohm Press, 2000.

Scammell, Henry. *The New Arthritis Breakthrough.* New York: M. Evans and Company, 1998.

Shlotzhauer, Tammi, et al., *Living with Rheumatoid Arthritis.* Baltimore: Johns Hopkins University Press, 1995.

Theodosakis, Jason, et al. *The Arthritis Cure: The Medical Miracle That Can Halt, Reverse, and May Even Cure Osteoarthritis.* New York: Griffin Trade Paperback, 1998.

Gout

Emmerson, Bryan, and Bruce Emmer. *Getting Rid of Gout: A Guide to Management and Prevention.* New York: Oxford University Press, 1996.

Schneiter, Jodi. *The Gout Hater's Cookbook: Recipes Lower in Purines.* Palm Coast, Fla.: Reachment Publications, 1999.

Fibromyalgia and Chronic Fatigue Syndrome

Goldberg, Burton. *Alternative Medicine Guide to Chronic Fatigue, Fibromyalgia and Environmental Illness.* Future Medicine Publishing, 1998.

Hammerly, Milton. *Fibromyalgia: The New Integrative Approach, How to Combine the Best of Traditional and Alternative Therapies.* Holbrook, Mass.: Adams Media Corporation, 2000.

Salt II, William B., and Edwin H. Season. *Fibromyalgia and the Mind, Body, Spirit Connection: 7 Steps for Living a Healthy Life with Widespread Muscular Pain and Fatigue.* Columbus, Ohio: Parkview Publishing, 2000.

Selli, Mari, Andrea Helm, and Paul D. Brown. *Alternative Treatments for Fibromyalgia and Chronic Fatigue Syndrome: Insights from Practitioners and Patients.* Alameda, Calif.: Hunter House, 1999.

Starlanyl, Devin J., and Mary Ellen Copeland, *Fibromyalgia & Chronic Myofascial Pain Syndrome: A Survival Manual.* Oakland: New Harbinger Publications, 1996.

Tendinitis/Bursitis

Hoffman, David. *Healthy Bones & Joints: A Natural Approach to Treating Arthritis, Osteoporosis, Tendinitis, Myalgia and Bursitis*. Pownal, Vt.: Storey Books, 2000.

Scott, W. Norman, et al. *Dr. Scott's Knee Book: Symptoms, Diagnosis and Treatment of Knee Problems, including Torn Cartilage, Ligament Damage, Arthritis, Tendinitis*. Fireside, 1996.

Natural Medicine

James LaValle, et al. *Natural Therapeutics Pocket Guide*. Hudson, Ohio: LexiComp, 2000.

Carol Newall, et al. *Herbal Medicines: A Guide for Health-Care Professionals*. London: Pharmaceutical Press, 1996

Ross Pelton, et al. *Drug-Induced Nutrient Depletion Handbook*. Hudson, Ohio: LexiComp, 1999.

Volker Schulz, et al., *Rational Phytotherapy*. New York: Springer-Verlag, 1998.

ORGANIZATIONS AND WEB SITES

General Medical and Alternative Medicine On-line Resources

www.altmed.com
www.altmedicine.com
www.health.harvard.edu
www.intelihealth.com
www.intramedicine.com
www.mayoclinic.com
www.medscape.com
www.nccam.nih.gov
www.nextpharmaceuticals.com
www.webmd.com
www.wellnessletter.com

Organizations

American Academy of Osteopathy
3500 DePauw Boulevard, Suite 1080
Indianapolis, IN 46268-1136
317-879-1881
www.academyofosteopathy.org

American Botanical Council
P.O. Box 201660
Austin, TX 78720
512-331-8868
Fax: 512-331-1924
www.healthworld.com/library/periodicals/journals/HerbalGram/
index.html

American Holistic Medical Association
6728 Old McLean Drive
McLean, VA 22101
703-556-9246
www.holisticmedicine.org

American Institute of Stress
124 Park Avenue
Yonkers, NY 10703
914-963-1200
www.stress.org

American College of Preventive Medicine
1660 L Street, NW
Washington, DC 20036
202-466-2044
www.acpm.org

Bastyr University of Natural Health Sciences
14500 Juanita Drive NE
Bothell, WA 98011
425-823-1300
Fax: 425-823-6222
www.bastyr.edu/index.html

Herb Research Foundation
1007 Pearl Street, Suite 200
Boulder, CO 80302
303-449-2265
www.herbs.org

National College of Naturopathic Medicine
049 SW Porter Street
Portland, OR 97201
503-499-4343
www.ncnm.edu

Townsend Letter for Doctors and Patients
911 Tyler Street
Port Townsend, WA 98368
360-385-6021
www.tldp.com

American Pain Society
4700 W. Lake Avenue
Glenview, IL 60025
847-375-4715
www.ampainsoc.org

Center for Medical Consumers
130 MacDougal Street
New York, NY 10012
212-674-7105
www.medicalconsumers.org

International Association for the Study of Pain
909 NE 43rd Street, Suite 306
Seattle, WA 98105
206-547-6409
www.halcyon.com/iasp

Laughter Works
P.O. Box 1076
Fair Oaks, CA 95628
916-863-1592
www.laughterworks.com

National Chronic Pain Outreach Association
7979 Old Georgetown Road, Suite 100
Bethesda, MD 20814-2429
310-652-4948

Public Citizens Health Research Group
1600 20th Street, NW
Washington, DC 20009
202-588-1000
www.citizen.org

Arthritis Foundation
National Office
1330 West Peachtree Street
Atlanta, Georgia 30309
404-872-7100
www.arthritis.org

Arthritis Resource Center
www.HealingWell.com/arthritis

The Johns Hopkins Arthritis Center
www.hopkins-arthritis.som.jhmi.edu

National Institute of Arthritis and Musculoskeletal and Skin Diseases
National Institutes of Health
Bethesda, MD 20892-2350
www.nih.gov/niams

National Library of Medicine's Medline Plus Health Information on
Gout and Pseudogout
www.nlm.nih.gov/medlineplus/goutandpseudogout.html

American College of Rheumatology's Factsheet on Gout
www.rheumatology.org/patients/factsheet/gout.html

The American Fibromyalgia Syndrome Association, Inc.
6380 E. Tanque Verde, Suite D
Tucson, AZ 85715
520-733-1570
www.afsafund.org

Fibromyalgia Network
P.O. Box 31750
Tucson, AZ 85715
800-853-2929
www.fmnetnews.com

The Oregon Fibromyalgia Foundation
www.myalgia.com

American Association for Chronic Fatigue Syndrome
c/o Harborview Medical Center
325 Ninth Avenue, Box 359780
Seattle, WA 98104
206-521-1932
www.aacfs.org

The Chronic Fatigue and Immune Disfunction Syndrome (CFIDS)
Association of America Inc.
P.O. Box 220398
Charlotte, NC 28222-0398
www.cfids.org

Chronic Fatigue Syndrome Electronic Newsletter
www.cfs-news.org

National Library of Medicine's Medline Plus Health Information on
Bursitis and Tendinitis
www.nlm.nih.gov/medlineplus/bursitis.html

American College of Rheumatology's Factsheet on Bursitis and Tendinitis
www.rheumatology.org/patients/factsheet/tendin.html

Notes

CHAPTER 4. COX-2 INHIBITORS: A REVOLUTION IN THE TREATMENT OF INFLAMMATION

1. J. R. Vane, Y. S. Bakhle, and R. M. Botting, "Cyclooxygenases 1 and 2," *Annu Rev Pharmacol Toxicol* 38 (1998): 97–120.

2. C. Larousse and G. Veyrac, "Clinical Data on Cox-1 and Cox-2 Inhibitors: What Possible Alerts in Pharmacovigilance?" *Therapie* 55, no. 1 (January/February 2000): 21–28.

3. K. Seibert et al., "Cox-2 Inhibitors: Is There Cause for Concern?" *Nat Med* 5, no. 6 (June 1999): 621–22.

4. T. J. Schnitzer, "Cyclooxygenase-2-specific Inhibitors: Are They Safe?" *American Journal of Medicine* 110, no. 1A (January 8, 2000): 46S–49S.

CHAPTER 5. THE COX-2 CONNECTION IN ALZHEIMER'S AND CANCER

1. G. Dannhardt and W. Kiefer, "Cyclooxygenase Inhibitors: Current Status and Future Prospects," *Eur J Med Chem* 36, no. 2 (February 2001): 109–26.

2. T. Kawamori et al., "Chemopreventive Activity of Celecoxib, a Specific Cyclooxygenase-2 Inhibitor, Against Colon Carcinogenesis," *Cancer Res* 58 (February 1998): 3, 409–12.

3. I. R. MacKenzie et al., "Non-steroidal Anti-inflammatory Drug Use and Alzheimer-type Pathology in Aging," *Neurol* 50 (1998): 986–90.

4. B. L. Flynn and K. A. Theesen, "Pharmacologic Management of Alzheimer's Disease," part 3 of "Non-steroidal Anti-inflammatory Drugs: Emerging Protective Evidence?" *Ann Pharmacother* 33, no. 7–8 (July/August 1999): 840–49.

5. J. C. Anthony et al., "Reduced Prevalence of AD in Users of NSAIDs and H2 Receptor Antagonists: The Cache County Study," *Neurology* 54, no. 11 (June 13, 2000): 2066–71.

6. B. L. Fiebich et al., "Effects of NSAIDs on IL-1beta-induced IL-6 mRNA and Protein Synthesis in Human Astrocytoma Cells," *NeuroReport* 7 (1996): 1209–13.

7. G. P. Lim et al., "Ibuprofen Suppresses Plaque Pathology and Inflammation in a Mouse Model for Alzheimer's Disease," *J Neurosci* 20 (2000): 5709–14.

8. J. L. Cummings et al., "Alzheimer's Disease: Etiologies, Pathophysiology, Cognitive Reserve, and Treatment Opportunities," *Neurology* 51, no.1, Supplement 1 (1998): S2–17.

9. J.C. Breitner et al., "Inverse Association of Anti-inflammatory Treatments and Alzheimer's Disease: Initial Results of a Co-twin Control Study," *Neurology* 44 (1994): 227–32.

10. I. Alafuzoff et al., "Lower Counts of Astroglia and Activated Microglia in Patients with Alzheimer's Disease with Regular Use of Non-steroidal Anti-inflammatory Drugs," *J Alzheimer's Dis* 2 (2000): 37–46.

11. W. F. Stewart et al., "Risk of Alzheimer's Disease and Duration of NSAID Use," *Neurology* 48, no. 3 (1997): 626–32.

12. J. Rogers et al., "Clinical Trial of Indomethacin in Alzheimer's Disease," *Neurology* 43, no. 8 (1993): 1609–11.

13. U. Abel, "Chemotherapy of Advanced Epithelial Cancer: A Critical Review," *Biomed Pharmacother* 46 (1992): 439–52.

14. P. Lichtenstein et al., "Environmental and Heritable Factors in the Causation of Cancer Analyses of Cohorts of Twins from Sweden, Denmark, and Finland," *New England Journal of Medicine* 343 (2000): 78–85.

15. R. N. Maric and K. K. Cheng, "Meat Intake, Heterocyclic Amines, and Colon Cancer," *American Journal of Gastroenterology* 95, no. 12 (December 2000): 3683–84.

16. W. J. Crinnion, "Environmental Medicine" part 1: "The Human Burden of Environmental Toxins and Their Common Health Effects," *Altern Med Rev* 5 (2000): 52–63.

17. The Centers for Disease Control and Prevention, "Trends in screening for colorectal cancer—United States, 1997 and 1999," *Journal of the American Medical Association* 285, no. 12 (March 28, 2001): 1570–71.

18. O. Gallo et al., "Cyclooxygenase-2 Pathway Correlates with VEGF Expression in Head and Neck Cancer. Implications for Tumor Angiogenesis and Metastasis," *Neoplasia* 3, no. 1 (January 2001): 53–61.

19. P. J. Bostrom et al., "Interferon-alpha Inhibits Cyclooxygenase-1 and Stimulates Cyclooxygenase-2 Expression in Bladder Cancer Cells in Vitro," *Urol Res.* 29, no. 1 (February 2001): 20–24.

20. X. H. Liu et al., "Inhibition of Cyclooxygenase-2 Suppresses Angiogenesis and the Growth of Prostate Cancer in Vivo," part 1, *J Urol* 164, no. 3 (September 2000): 820–25.

21. P. M. Lynch, "Cox-2 Inhibition in Clinical Cancer Prevention," *Oncology* no. 3, Supplement 5 (March 15, 2001): 21–26.

22. M. Li et al., "Induction of Apoptosis in Colon Cancer Cells by Cyclooxygenase-2 Inhibitor NS398 through a Cytochrome c-dependent Pathway," *Clin Cancer Res* 7, no. 4 (April 2001): 1010–16.

23. T. Kawamori et al., "Chemopreventive Activity of Celecoxib, a Specific Cyclooxygenase-2 Inhibitor, Against Colon Carcinogenesis," *Cancer Res* 58, no. 3 (February 1, 1998): 409–12.

24. S. Tomozawa et al., "Cyclooxygenase-2 Overexpression Correlates with Tumour Recurrence, Especially Haematogenous Metastasis, of Colorectal Cancer," *Br J Cancer* 83, no. 3 (August 2000): 324–28.

25. B. A. Erickson et al., "The Effect of Selective Cyclooxygenase Inhibitors on Intestinal Epithelial Cell Mitogenesis," *J Surg Res* 81, no. 1 (January 1999): 101–07.

26. G. Steinbach et al., "The Effect of Celecoxib, a Cyclooxygenase-2 Inhibitor, in Familial Adenomatous Polyposis," *New England Journal of Medicine* 342, no. 26 (June 29, 2000): 1946–52.

27. S. Ota et al., "Colorectal Cancer and Non-steroidal Anti-inflammatory Drugs," *Acta Pharmacol Sin* 21, no. 5 (May 2000): 391–95.

28. C. S. Williams et al., "Host Cyclooxygenase-2 Modulates Carcinoma Growth," *J Clin Invest* 105, no. 11 (June 2000): 1589–94.

CHAPTER 6. NATURAL COX-2 INHIBITORS AND OTHER NATURAL REMEDIES

1. J. Wasik, "The Truth About Herbal Supplements," *Consumer's Digest*, July/August 1999, 75–76, 78–79.

2. Y. C. Chen et al., "Wogonin, Baicalin, and Baicalein Inhibition of Inducible Nitric Oxide Synthase and Cyclooxygenase-2 Gene Expressions Induced by Nitric Oxide Synthase Inhibitors and Lipopolysaccharide," *Biochem Pharmacol* 61, no. 11 (June 1, 2001): 1417–27.

3. E. S. Johnson et al., "Efficacy of Feverfew as Prophylactic Treatment of Migraine," *British Medical Journal* 291 (1985): 569–73.

4. C. A. Newall et al., pp. 119–21.

5. M. J. Biggs et al., "Platelet Aggregation in Patients Using Feverfew for Migraine," *Lancet* 2, no. 8301 (1982): 776.

6. H. Bliddal et al., "A Randomized, Placebo-controlled, Cross-over Study of Ginger Extracts and Ibuprofen in Osteoarthritis," *Osteoarthritis Cartilage* 8, no. 1 (January 2000): 9–12.

7. A. Bordia, S. K. Verma, and K. C. Srivastava, "Effect of Ginger (*Zingiber officinale* Rose) and Fenugreek (*Trigonella foenumgraecum* L.) on Blood Lipids, Blood Sugar and Platelet Aggregation in Patients with Coronary Artery Disease," *Prostaglandins Leukot Essent Fatty Acids* 56, no. 5 (May 1997): 379–84.

8. T. M. Haqqi et al., "Prevention of Collagen-induced Arthritis in Mice by a Polyphenolic Fraction from Green Tea," *Proc Natl Acad Sci USA* 96, no. 8 (April 1999): 4524–29.

9. V. M. Hegarty, H. M. May, and K. T. Khaw, "Tea Drinking and Bone Mineral Density in Older Women," *Am J Clin Nutr* 71, no. 4 (April 2000): 1003–07.

10. M. A. Kelm et al., "Antioxidant and Cyclooxygenase Inhibitory Phenolic Compounds from *Ocimum Sanctum* Linn," *Phytomedicine* 7, no. 1 (March 2000): 7–13.

11. B. Obertreis et al., "Anti-inflammatory Effect of *Urtica dioica folia* Extract in Comparison to Caffeic Malic Acid," *Arzneim-Forsch/Drug Res* 46, no. 1(January 1996): 52–56.

12. M. A. Kelm, M. G. Nair, and G. M. Strasburg, "Antioxidant and Cyclooxygenase Inhibitory Phenolic Compounds from *Ocimum sanctum* Linn," *Phytomedicine* 7, no. 1 (March 2000): 7–13.

13. M. Benito et al., "Labiatae Allergy: Systemic Reactions Due to Ingestion of Oregano and Thyme," *Ann Allergy Asthma Immunol* 76, no. 5 (May 1996): 416–18.

14. J. M. Snow, "*Curcuma Longa* L. (Zingiberaceae)," *Protocol Journal of Botanical Medicine* 1, no. 2 (Autumn 1995): 43–46.

15. R. S. Ramsewak, D. L. DeWitt, and M. G. Nair, "Cytotoxicity, Antioxidant and Anti-inflammatory Activities of Curcumins I-III from *Curcuma longa*," *Phytomedicine* 7, no. 4 (July 2000): 303–08.

16. T. Uchiyama et al., "Anti-ulcer Effect of Extract from Phellodendri Cortex," *Yakugaku Zasshi* 109, no. 9 (September 1989): 672–76.

17. A. L. Vaz, "Double-blind Clinical Evaluation of the Relative Efficacy of Ibuprofen and Glucosamine Sulfate in the Management of Osteoarthrosis of the Knee in Out-patients," *Curr Med Res Opin* 8, no. 3 (1982): 145–49.

18. H. Muller-Fassbender et al., "Glucosamine Sulfate Compared to Ibuprofen in Osteoarthritis of the Knee," *Osteoarthritis and Cartilage* 2, no. 1 (1994): 61–69.

19. G. X. Qui et al., "Efficacy and Safety of Glucosamine Sulfate Versus Ibuprofen in Patients with Knee Osteoarthritis," *Arzneimittelforschung* 48, no. 5 (May 1998): 469–74.

20. V. R. Pipitone, "Chondroprotection with Chondroitin Sulfate," *Drugs Exp Clin Res* 17, no. 1 (1991): 3–7.

21. G. S. Kelly, "The Role of Glucosamine Sulfate and Chondroitin Sulfates in the Treatment of Degenerative Joint Disease," *Altern Med Rev* 3, no. 1 (February 1998): 27–39.

22. L. Bucci and G. Poor, "Efficacy and Tolerability of Oral Chondroitin Sulfate as a Symptomatic Slow-acting Drug for Osteoarthritis (SYSADOA) in the Treatment of Knee Osteoarthritis," *Osteoarthritis Cartilage* 6, Supplement A (May 1998): 31–36.

23. P. R. Bradley, ed., *The British Herbal Compendium*, vol. 1 (London: British Herbal Medicine Association, 1992), 224–26.

24. P. Geusens et al., "Long-term Effect of Omega-3 Fatty Acid Supplementation in Active Rheumatoid Arthritis. A 12-Month, Double-blind, Controlled Study," *Arthritis Rheum* 37, no. 6 (June 1994): 824–29.

CHAPTER 7. CURRENT TREATMENT OPTIONS

1. H. P. Ammon, "Salai Guggal-*Boswellia serrata*: From an Herbal Medicine to a Non-redox Inhibitor of Leukotriene Biosynthesis," *Eur J Med Res* 1, no. 8 (May 1996): 369–70.

2. H. P. Ammon et al., "Inhibition of Leukotriene B4 Formation in Rat Peritoneal

Neutrophils by an Ethanolic Extract of the Gum Resin Exudate of *Boswellia serrata*," *Planta Med* 57, no. 3 (June 1991): 203–07.

3. R. Maffei Facino et al., "Regeneration of Endogenous Antioxidants, Ascorbic Acid, Alpha Tocopherol, by the Oligomeric Procyanide Fraction of *Vitis vinifera* L: ESR Study. *Boll Chim Farm* 136, no. 4 (1997): 340–44.

4. M. Jonadet et al., "Anthocyanosides Extracted from *Vitis vinifera, Vaccinium myrtillus* and *Pinus maritimus.* I. Elastase-inhibiting Activities in Vitro. II. Compared Angioprotective Activities in Vivo," *J Pharm Belg* 38, no. 1 (1983): 41–46.

5. E. N. Frankel et al., "Inhibition of Oxidation of Human Low-density Lipoprotein by Phenolic Substances in Red Wine," *Lancet* 341, no. 8843 (1993): 454–57.

6. H. P. Ammon et al., "Mechanism of Anti-inflammatory Actions of Curcumin and Boswellic Acids," *J Ethnopharmacol* 38 (1993): 113.

7. K. C. Srivastava et al., "Curcumin, A Major Component of Food Spice Turmeric *(Curcuma longa)* Inhibits Aggregation and Alters Eicosanoid Metabolism in Human Blood Platelets," *Prostaglandins Leukot Essent Fatty Acids* 52, no. 4 (April 1995): 223–27.

8. J. M. Snow, "*Curcuma Longa* L. (Zingiberaceae)," *Protocol Journal of Botanical Medicine* 1, no. 2 (Autumn 1995): 43–46.

9. L. G. Miller, "Herbal Medicinals: Selected Clinical Considerations Focusing on Known or Potential Drug-Herb Interactions," *Arch Intern Med* 158, no. 20 (November 1998): 2200–11.

10. K. S. Vaddadi, "The Use of Gamma-linolenic Acid and Linoleic Acid to Differentiate Between Temporal Lobe Epilepsy and Schizophrenia," *Prostaglandins Med* 6, no. 4 (April 1981): 375–79.

11. K. C. Dines et al., "Nerve Function in Galactosaemic Rats: Effects of Evening Primrose Oil and Doxazosin," *Eur J Pharmacol* 281, no. 3 (1995): 303–09.

12. J. P. De La Cruz et al., "Effect of Evening Primrose Oil on Platelet Aggregation in Rabbits Fed an Atherogenic Diet," *Thromb Res* 87, no. 1 (July 1997): 1414–19.

13. L. G. Miller, "Herbal Medicinals: Selected Clinical Considerations Focusing on Known or Potential Drug-Herb Interactions," *Arch Intern Med* 158, no. 20 (November 1998): 2200–11.

14. K. S. Vaddadi, "The Use of Gamma-linolenic Acid and Linoleic Acid to Differentiate Between Temporal Lobe Epilepsy and Schizophrenia," *Prostaglandins Med* 6, no. 4 (April 1981): 375–79.

15. J. M. Pujalte et al., "Double-blind Clinical Evaluation of Oral Glucosamine Sulfate in the Basic Treatment of Osteoarthrosis," *Curr Med Res Opin* 7, no. 2 (1980): 110–14.

16. R. Rizzo, "Calcium, Sulfur and Zinc Distribution in Normal and Arthritic Articular Equine Cartilage: A Synchrotron Radiation Induced X-ray Emission Study," *Journal of Experimental Zoology* 237, no. 1 (September 1995): 82–86.

17. C. di Padova, "S-adenosylmethionine in the Treatment of Osteoarthritis. Review of the Clinical Studies," *American Journal of Medicine* 83, no. 5A (November 20, 1987): 60–65.

18. H. P. Ammon, "Salai Guggal-*Boswellia serrata:* From an Herbal Medicine to a

Non-redox Inhibitor of Leukotriene Biosynthesis," *Eur J Med Res* 1, no. 8 (May 1996): 369–370.

19. H. P. Ammon et al., "Inhibition of Leukotriene B4 Formation in Rat Peritoneal Neutrophils by an Ethanolic Extract of the Gum Resin Exudate of *Boswellia serrata*," *Planta Med* 57, no. 3 (June 1991): 203–207.

20. R. Maffei Facino et al., "Regeneration of Endogenous Antioxidants, Ascorbic Acid, Alpha Tocopherol, by the Oligomeric Procyanide Fraction of *Vitis vinifera* L: ESR Study," *Boll Chim Farm* 136, no. 4 (1997): 340–44.

21. M. Jonadet et al., "Anthocyanosides Extracted from Vitis vinifera, *Vaccinium myrtillus* and *Pinus maritimus*. I. Elastase-inhibiting Activities in Vitro. II. Compared Angioprotective Activities in Vivo," *J Pharm Belg* 38, no. 1 (1983): 41–46.

22. E. N. Frankel et al., "Inhibition of Oxidation of Human Low-density Lipoprotein by Phenolic Substances in Red Wine," *Lancet* 341, no. 8843 (1993): 454–57.

23. L. G. Miller, "Herbal Medicinals: Selected Clinical Considerations Focusing on Known or Potential Drug-Herb Interactions," *Arch Intern Med* 158. no. 20 (November 1998): 2200–11.

24. K. S. Vaddadi, "The Use of Gamma-linolenic Acid and Linoleic Acid to Differentiate Between Temporal Lobe Epilepsy and Schizophrenia," *Prostaglandins Med* 6, no. 4 (April 1981): 375–79.

25. K. C. Dines et al., "Nerve Function in Galactosaemic Rats: Effects of Evening Primrose Oil and Doxazosin," *Eur J Pharmacol* 281, no. 3 (1995): 303–09.

26. J. P. De La Cruz et al., "Effect of Evening Primrose Oil on Platelet Aggregation in Rabbits Fed an Atherogenic Diet," *Thromb Res* 87, no. 1 (July 1997): 1414–19.

27. L. G. Miller, "Herbal Medicinals: Selected Clinical Considerations Focusing on Known or Potential Drug-Herb Interactions," *Arch Intern Med* 158, no. 20 (November 1998): 2200–11.

28. K. S. Vaddadi, "The Use of Gamma-linolenic Acid and Linoleic Acid to Differentiate Between Temporal Lobe Epilepsy and Schizophrenia," *Prostaglandins Med* 6, no. 4 (April 1981): 375–79.

29. M. A. Kelm et al., "Antioxidant and Cyclooxygenase Inhibitory Phenolic Compounds from *Ocimum sanctum* Linn," *Phytomedicine* 7, no. 1 (March 2000): 7–13.

30. F. Brinker, *Herb Contraindications and Drug Interactions* (Sandy, Ore.: Eclectic Institute, 1997), 70.

31. J. M. Pujalte et al., "Double-blind Clinical Evaluation of Oral Glucosamine Sulfate in the Basic Treatment of Osteoarthrosis," *Curr Med Res Opin* 7, no. 2 (1980): 110–14.

32. R. Rizzo, "Calcium, Sulfur and Zinc Distribution in Normal and Arthritic Articular Equine Cartilage: A Synchrotron Radiation Induced X-ray Emission Study," *Journal of Experimental Zoology* 237, no. 1 (September 1995): 82–86.

33. C. di Padova, "S-adenosylmethionine in the Treatment of Osteoarthritis. Review of the Clinical Studies," *Am J Med* 83, no. 5A (November 20, 1987): 60–65.

34. B. Obertreis et al., "Anti-inflammatory Effect of *Urtica dioica folia* Extract in Comparison to Caffeic Malic Acid," *Arzneim-Forsch/Drug Res* 46, no. 1 (January 1996): 52–56.

35. S. Cunningham-Rundles et al., "Nutrition and the Immune System of the Gut," *Nutrition* 14, no. 7–8 (July 1998): 573–79.

36. A. L. Miller, "Therapeutic Considerations of L-glutamine: A Review of the Literature," *Altern Med Rev* 4, no. 4 (August 1999): 239–48.

37. M. Gonzalez et al., "Hypoglycemic Activity of Olive Leaf," *Planta Med* 58, no. 6 (December 1992): 513–15.

38. B. Fehri et al., "Hypotension, Hypoglycemia and Hypouricemia Recorded After Repeated Administration of Aqueous Leaf Extract of *Olea europaea* L.," *J Pharm Belg* 49, no. 2 (March/April 1994): 101–08.

39. A. Petroni et al., "Inhibition of Platelet Aggregation and Eicosanoid Production by Phenolic Components of Olive Oil," *Thromb Res* 78, no. 2 (April 15, 1995): 151–60.

40. J. B. LaValle et al., *Natural Therapeutics Pocket Guide* (Hudson, Ohio: LexiComp, 2000), 483–84, 404–5.

41. R. Aquino et al., "Plant Metabolites. Structure and in Vitro Antiviral Activity of Quinovic Acid Glycosides from *Uncaria tomentosa* and *Guettarda platypoda*," *J Nat Prod* 52, no. 4 (1989): 679–85.

42. S. M. de Matta et al., "Alkaloids and Procyanidins of an *Uncaria* sp. from Peru," *Farmaco* (Sci) 31, no. 7 (1976): 527–35.

43. R. Aquino et al., "Plant Metabolites. New Compounds and Anti-inflammatory Activity of *Uncaria tomentosa*," *J Nat Prod* 54, no. 2 (1981): 453–59.

44. G. Ionescu et al., "Oral Citrus Seed Extract," *J Orthomolecula Med* 5, no. 3 (1990): 72–74.

45. G. W. Bray, "Hypochlorhydria of Asthma in Childhood," *Quarterly Journal of Medicine* 24 (January 1931): 181–89.

Index

(Note: Page numbers in *italic* indicate charts.)

acetaminophen, 4, 15
  contraindications, 90
  as treatment for Alzheimer's disease, 60
  as treatment for osteoarthritis pain, 90
acupressure, for pain relief, 123–124
acupuncture, for pain relief, 117
adaptive immune system, 8
aerobic exercise, 89
affirmation, to combat negative thinking, 131–132
Alexander Technique, 134
allergies
  to food, 40, 114
  to medications and chemicals, 45, 81
  to oregano, 77
allopurinol, 103
alternative medicine.
  See complementary health care
altruism, and role in pain relief, 125–126
Alzheimer's disease
  Cox-2 inhibitors and, 56–61
Alzheimer's Disease Anti-Inflammatory
  Prevention Trial (ADAPT), 60
American College of Rheumatology, 46
anatomy, 18–29
angiogenesis (formation of new blood
  vessels), 54, 62–63
antibiotics
  and chronic fatigue syndrome, 49
  and dysbiosis, 106–107
antibodies, 8–9
antihistamines, contraindications for
  exercise, 137
antimalarial drugs, as treatment for rheumatoid arthritis, 98
antioxidants, 83

antirheumatic drugs, 98
apoptosis, 56, 61
arthritis, 30–40. *See also* osteoarthritis
  and rheumatoid arthritis
  gout, connection to, 41
  self-help pain reduction program,
    141–142
Arthritis Foundation, 113, 141–142
  diet guidelines of, 114
arthrodesis, 95
arthroplasty, 95
arthroscopy, 95
aspirin, 4, 15, 53
  and Alzheimer's disease, 60
  contraindications, 94, 137
  in treatment of bursitis, 106
  in treatment of rheumatoid arthritis, 98
autogenic phrases, 124
autoimmune response, 25, 37
autonomic nervous system, 9–10
Azulfidine-EN-tabs (sulfasalazine), 99
baikal skullcap, 73
Baltimore Longitudinal Study of Aging,
  60
batherapy, 142
B-cells, 8–9
Bethesda Pain Control Program, 143–144
biofeedback, for pain relief, 117
body fat, measuring, 36
body mass index, 36
body temperature, role in pain relief,
  126–127
"bodymind," 5, 51.
  See also "mind-body connection"
bones, 20–22
  infections, 24

breast-feeding and natural immunity, 8
breathing, deep, for pain relief, 112, 124
bursitis, 28, 47–48
    treatment of, 105–106

caffeine, effect of, on pain, 129–130
cancer
    and angiogenesis, 54
    and Cox-2 inhibitors, 61–63
capsaicin, 127
cardiac muscle, 20
celecoxib (Celebrex), 50–52, 62
central nervous system, 7–8
chemotherapy, connection to gout, 41
cherry juice concentrate, in treating gout,
    104
Chinese herbal medicine, 138–139
chiropractic therapy, 140
chondroitin sulfate, 80–81
chronic fatigue syndrome, 43, 49
clinics, pain, 120, 124
coffee
    effect of, on pain, 129–130
    substitutes for, 130
colchicine, 103, 104
cold, for pain relief, 88, 118
colon polyps, 62
complementary health care, 6, 14–15
    with fibromyalgia, 105
connective tissue diseases, 25
corticosteroids, 90, 91, 98, 104
counterirritants, 94
Cox-1, 52, 57, 58, 61
Cox 2, 51, 52, 58–59, 61
Cox-1 inhibitors, 78–79
Cox-2 inhibitors, 5, 15, 50–55, 94
    herbal, 68–79
    other natural remedies, 79–85
    as treatment for Alzheimer's disease
        and cancer, 56–66
    as treatment for rheumatoid arthritis,
        98
cramps, 27
cyclooxygenase, 4, 54, 58, 62, 75

cyclophosphamide (Cytoxan), 99
cyclosporin, 99
cytoprotective agents, 93
Cytoxan (cyclophosphamide), 99
cytotoxic T-cells, 8–9

deep breathing, for pain relief, 112
depression, 45–46
diabetes, association with pseudogout, 42
diet, 83, 114. See also nutrition
"differential diagnosis," 34
diuretics, contraindications for exercise,
    137
drug-free pain control, 144
drugs. See also nonsteroidal anti-
        inflammatory drugs and specific drugs
    development of, 63–64, 65
    discovery of, 65
    overuse of, for pain, 137
    for pain relief, 127
    psychoactive, 13
    standardization of, 65–66
    for treatment of inflammation, 15–16
dry eye syndrome, 106
dysbiosis, 40, 44
    treatment of, 106–108

emotional trauma and connection to
        disease, 11
endogenous factors, 5
endorphins, 12
    in pain relief, 112, 118, 123, 128,
        131, 144
endurance exercise, 88–89
environmental toxins, 49
epinephrine, 9, 10
essential oils, 83
exercise, 16, 23, 45, 127
    aerobic, 89
    endurance, 88–89
    isometric, 89
    and medications, 137
    for muscle strengthening, 88–89
    for osteoarthritis, 141

as pain relief, 88–89, 114, 142–143
    in treatment of bursitis, 106
    in treatment of fibromyalgia, 104–105
    in treatment of rheumatoid arthritis, 97
    value of pacing yourself, 134
    walking as, 144–145
    water workouts as, 89
exercise instructors, for pain relief, 116
exogenous factors, 5

familial adenomatous polyposis (FAP), 62
fasting, in treatment of gout, 103
fatigue
    with fibromyalgia, 104
    with rheumatoid arthritis, 96
Feldenkrais Technique, 135
feverfew, 73
fibromyalgia, 27, 43–47
    treatment of, 104–105
fish oil, 81–82
foot pain, massage for, 121
free radicals, 58–59, 83
frozen shoulder, 29
functional integration, 135

"generally regarded as safe" (GRAS) list,
    72
genetic factors in onset of osteoarthritis,
    32, 35
ginger, 75
"glove anesthesia," 136
glucosamine, 79–81
gold salt therapy, 99
gout, 41–43
    contraindications for drug therapies,
        103
    diet as a factor in, 103
    natural therapies for, 104
    treatment of, with drugs, 103

habits, breaking pain-related, 135–136
health insurance coverage, 15, 73
heat, for pain relief, 118
helper cells, 9
helping others, role in pain relief, 125–126

herbal remedies, 68–79, 92–93. See also
    natural remedies
    Chinese, 138–139
Hippocrates and mind-body connection, 6
histamine, 3–4
hormones, 12
hot chili peppers, for pain relief, 127
hydrochloride, 79
hypnosis, 12
    for pain relief, 118

ibuprofen, 4, 15, 58
    as treatment for Alzheimer's disease,
        58, 59
    as treatment for rheumatoid arthritis,
        98
immune response, 8, 40, 58, 114
    abnormalities, 44
    in dysbiosis, 106, 107
    influence on, by hypnosis, 12
    influence on, by stress, 11–12
immune system, 6–9
immunological organs, 7
immunosuppressive drugs, 98, 99
inflammation, 3–17, 23–24, 25, 37, 41
    absence of, 44
    in Alzheimer's disease, 57–58
    in association with Cox-2 inhibitors, 51
    in dysbiosis, 106
    reduced by rest, 97
interferons, 9, 12
interleukins, 9, 12
involuntary muscles, 18
iron in tissues, association with
    pseudogout, 42
isometric exercise, 89

joints, 21–22
    diseases of, 25
    infections in, 24

kava kava, in treatment of fibromyalgia,
    105
ketoprofen, 4, 15

laughter, for pain relief, 122, 132–133
"leaky gut" syndrome, 40, 106
life expectancy, effect on, of health, 23
lifestyle changes, effect on, of health, 17
liver damage, protection from, 93
lumbago, osteopathy as a treatment for, 139
lymphocytes, 7, 8, 12
lymphoid organs, 7

MRI. See magnetic resonance imaging
magnetic resonance imaging (MRI), 24
malignancies, causes of, 61
massage
    for pain relief, 113, 121, 130
    self-massage, for neck pain, 141
mast cells, 3
medications and exercise, 137
medicinal plants (chart), 70
memory of immune system, 8
menopause and gout, 41
menthol gel, use in massage for pain
    relief, 130
methotrexate, 99
migraines, 45
milk thistle, 93
mind-body. See also "bodymind"
    connection, 6, 10–15, 122–123
    techniques, 16
motivation, role of, in pain control, 136
movement
    Alexander Technique, 134
    Feldenkrais Technique, 135
muscles, 18–20, 22
muscle-strengthening exercise, 88–89
musculoskeletal system, 21–22
    disorders of, 23, 25
    problems, 26–29
    treatment of problems, 24
music, for pain relief, 131
myotherapy, 143

NSAIDs. See nonsteroidal
    anti-inflammatory drugs
naprosyn, 98

naproxen, 4, 15, 52
narcotic drugs, 128
National Center for Complementary and
    Alternative Medicine (NCCAM),
    15, 72
National Institute on Aging (NIA), 60
natural immunity, and breast-feeding, 8
Natural Killer (NK) cells, 8–9
natural remedies, 16. See also herbal
    remedies and nondrug treatment
    methods
    for bursitis, 106
    in conjunction with non-narcotic
        drugs, 128
    for gout, 104
    product quality issues of, 83–86
neck pain, self-massage for, 141
negative influences on health, 123
negative thinking
    influence of pets on, 122
    motivation and effect on, 136
    use of affirmation to combat, 131
nervous system. See central nervous system
neuropathic pain, 110
neurotransmitters, 9, 12, 19, 94
newborn children and natural immunity, 8
Nexrutine, 79, 85
nociceptive pain, 110
nondrug treatment methods, 88–90.
    See also herbal remedies
    and natural remedies
non-narcotic drugs, 127–128
nonsteroidal anti-inflammatory drugs
    (NSAIDs), 4–5, 15, 52–53
    adverse effects of/contraindications
        for, 91, 107
    and Alzheimer's disease, 56–61
    in treatment of bursitis, 106
    in treatment of gout, 104
    in treatment of osteoarthritis, 91, 93
    in treatment of rheumatoid arthritis, 98
norepinephine, 9, 10
nutrient absorption in dysbiosis, 106
nutrition, 16, 49. See also diet

nutritional supplements, 137
   for dysbiosis, 107–108
   for fibromyalgia, 105
   for osteoarthritis, *92*
   for rheumatoid arthritis, *101–102*
nutritionists, for pain relief, 116

obesity
   as a cause of osteoarthritis, 32, 35, 113
   as risk factor for gout, 41
Office of Alternative Medicine (OAM), 72
omega-6 and omega-3 fatty acids, 81–82
   anti-inflammatory effect, 82
oregano, 77
osteoarthritis, 32–36
   and back pain, 141
   disease-modifying drugs for
      osteoarthritis (DMOADs), 96
   nutritional supplements for treating, *92*
   treatment options, 87–91, 93–96
osteopathy, 139
osteoporosis, 96, 99
osteotomy, 95

PNI. *See* psychoneuroimmunology
pacing yourself, for pain control, 134
pain
   in bursitis, 47–48
   with chronic fatigue syndrome, 49
   in fibromyalgia, 45
   management of, 109–145
   with osteoarthritis, 88
   use of exercise to control, 97
Pain Erasure (myotherapy), 143
parasympathetic nervous system, 9–10
penicillamine, 99
pets, for pain relief, 122
phellodendron, 79
physical therapists, for pain relief, 116
phytomedicines (herbal supplements), 68
placebo, role in pain relief, 128–129
plant sterolins, 100
polyps, treatment of colon, 62
positive attitude

   affirmation as a tool to express, 131
   and effect on motivation, 136
   and pain relief, 115
   and rheumatoid arthritis, 96
positive influences on health, *123*
prayer, for pain relief, 133
Prednisone, 98
Progressive Muscle Relaxation (PMR),
   119, 124
prostaglandins
   decreased production of, 61, 75
   defined, 58–59
   role of, in inflammation, 4, 52
pseudogout, 42–43
psychogenic pain, 110
psychological factors
   and fibromyalgia, 105
   and pain, 13
   and rheumatoid arthritis, 96
psychoneuroimmunology (PNI), 5, 6–7,
   10–14
psychosocial factors, effect on immune
   system response, 12

qi, 138–139

range-of-motion exercise, 88–89, 97
reflexology, 139
relaxation tapes, 124
repetitive motion, 47
repetitive strain disorder, 27
rest, as a factor in treating rheumatoid
   arthritis, 97. *See also* sleep
resurfacing, 95
Reye's Syndrome, 81
rheumatoid arthritis, 4, 25, 33, 37–40
   nutritional supplements, *101–102*
   treatment, 96–100
rheumatoid factor, 39
rofecoxib (Vioxx), 51–52
rosemary, 77

salicylic acid. *See* aspirin
secondary arthritis, 33

self-help
    program for arthritis, 141–142
    techniques for pain control, 111
self-hypnosis, for pain relief, 118
self-massage for neck pain, 141
sex, as a pain reliever, 112
skeletal muscles, 19
sleep. *See also* rest
    disturbances, 44, 49
    effect of body temperature on, 126–127
    with fibromyalgia, 105
    in pain relief, 117
smoking
    effect of quitting, on pain, 126
    as risk factor, 40
smooth muscle, 20
spas, 140
splints, to treat rheumatoid arthritis, 97
sprains, 26
standardization of herbal products, 84–86
stress
    bath to reduce, 142
    biofeedback for, 117
    and chronic fatigue syndrome, 49
    elimination of, with Feldenkrais
        Technique, 135
    and fibromyalgic pain, 45
    and immune system, 11–12, 13
    and nutrient depletion, 16
    oxidative, 83
    and pain, 116
sulfasalazine (Azulfidine-EN-tabs), 99
suppressor cells, 9
surgery
    as treatment for osteoarthritis, 94
    as treatment for rheumatoid arthritis,
        100
swimming, for pain relief, 142–143
sympathetic nervous system, 9
synthetic Cox-2 inhibitors, 51

tai chi, for osteoarthritis, 141
tapes, relaxation, 124
T-cells, 8–9

tendinitis, 27
therapeutic ratio, 64
therapeutic touch, 129
topical treatments for osteoarthritis, 94
tranquilizers, contraindications for
        exercise, 137
transcutaneous electrical nerve stimulation
        (TENS), 111
transdermal capability of oregano, 77
treatment options for inflammation and
        pain, 87–108
trigger points, 43
tumor growth, reduction of, 62–63
tumor-necrosis factor, 100
turmeric, 78
Twelve-Step Program for Coping with
        Chronic Pain, 120

ulcer complications, with Cox-2 drugs, 54
United States, herbal use in, 71–73
United States Pharmacopoeia (USP), 72
uric acid, 41, 42, 103

vacation, for pain relief, 140
Vioxx (rofecoxib), 50–52
viscosupplementation, 94
vitamin E as antioxidant, 83
vitamins and pain, 137.
        See also nutritional supplements
voluntary muscles, 18
volunteering, and role in pain relief,
        125–126

walking, for pain relief, 144–145
warmth, as pain relief, 88
water workouts, 89
weight control, 113, 114
white blood cells, 4, 7
willow bark, 81
workplace, pain relief in, 115

X rays, 24, 39, 42

yoga, for osteoarthritis, 141